Music and Dyslexia
Opening New Doors

EDITED BY

T.R. MILES
Professor Emeritus of Psychology,
University of Wales, Bangor

AND

JOHN WESTCOMBE
Adviser in Music Education and Careers

Consultant in Dyslexia
PROFESSOR MARGARET SNOWLING
University of York

W

WHURR PUBLISHERS
LONDON AND PHILADELPHIA

Chapter 3 © Violet Brand
Chapter 5 © Caroline Oldfield
Chapter 11 © Jacob Wiltshire
Chapter 20 © Margaret Hubicki
All other material © 2001 Whurr Publishers Ltd

First published 2001 by Whurr Publishers Ltd
19b Compton Terrace, London N1 2UN, England and
325 Chestnut Street, Philadelphia PA 19106, USA

Reprinted 2002 and 2004

British Library Cataloguing in Publication Data
A catalogue record for this book is available from the British
Library.

ISBN 1 86156 205 5

Printed and bound in the UK by Athenaeum Press Ltd,
Gateshead, Tyne & Wear

Music and Dyslexia

Contents

Contributors

Gill Backhouse is a chartered psychologist and honorary lecturer in the Department of Human Communication Science, University College, London. She works with dyslexic children and adults, helping to identify their strengths and to find a positive way of dealing with their difficulties.

Paula Bishop is currently finishing a Master's degree at the Royal Academy of Music, specializing in singing. She was awarded a BA Honours in Music from Oxford University while maintaining her vocal studies. Her operatic interests began when she played Flora in Britten's *The Turn of the Screw* (Scottish Opera) and her concert repertoire ranges from Renaissance to contemporary music. Paula is at present furthering her teaching interests, specializing in dyslexia, and has just started doctoral research into dyslexia and music alongside her singing career.

Violet Brand has been involved with the teaching of dyslexic children and adults for many years. She first became aware of the difficulties that dyslexics have with music in the 1960s – and has been learning more about them and ways of helping ever since. Her husband is a professional musician, so music and dyslexia meet in their house.

Nigel Clarke studied composition with Paul Patterson at the Royal Academy of Music, where he won many awards including the Queen's Commendation for Excellence. He has held a range of appointments including young composer in residence of the Hong Kong Academy for Performing Arts, associate composer to YCAT (Young Concert Artists' Trust), composition and contemporary music tutor at the Royal Academy of Music, and is currently composer in residence to the Black Dyke Mills Band. Nigel's music is performed extensively both nationally and internationally, and this includes both concerts and broadcasts. He has written two feature film scores to date – *Jinnah* and *The Little Vampire*. He is at present Head of Brass, Wind and Percussion and on the composition staff at the London College of Music and Media.

Janet Coker is a professional singer. She reports that from a very early age, long before she learned to read, she sang along with all the operatic arias that she heard on the radio. She was in her thirties before she discovered that she was dyslexic. She found it a source of great joy to know that she was not 'stupid', and that her dyslexia explained many of the difficulties that she had encountered when growing up. She has pursued a singing career in operas and operettas on the concert platform and on radio and television.

Diana Ditchfield studied piano and singing at the Royal Irish Academy of Music and at the University of Limerick. She has taught English and music in schools in England and Ireland and now works mainly at the Limerick Municipal School of Music.

Sylvia Gilpin is a sociologist and amateur flute and piano player. A parent of a dyslexic child, she is a member of the Campden Dyslexia Support Group and secretary to the British Dyslexia Association's Music Committee.

Margaret Hubicki is a past professor at the Royal Academy of Music and is the present consultant for *Music in the Community*. She is the originator of the text and materials of *Colour-Staff*.

Michael Lea is a double bass player. After joining the BBC Training Orchestra in Bristol in 1968 he went on to hold positions in the CBSO and the BBC Concert Orchestra. Since 1979 he has been a freelance principal bass player working in and around London. He has played in over 250 films and has taken part in many famous recordings. Between 1981 and 1988 he taught at the Guildhall School of Music, leaving in order to home-educate his children.

Tim Miles is Professor Emeritus of Psychology at the University of Wales, Bangor, and has published many books and papers on dyslexia and other topics. As a 'cellist he rates himself as 'decidedly amateur'.

Sheila Oglethorpe studied piano, 'cello and singing at the Royal Academy of Music. She has taught class and instrumental music and still teaches piano and theory at Salisbury Cathedral School. Her book, *Instrumental Music for Dyslexics: A Teaching Handbook,* was published in 1996. She lectures on the ABRSM Certificate of Teaching course.

Caroline Oldfield was a professional flute player who contributed to *Pan* (the journal of the British Flute Society) in 1987. We have obtained permission from *Pan* to reproduce the paper, but despite all our efforts we have been unable to trace her address.

Helen Poole was a keen musician at secondary school and was diagnosed as being 'dyscalculic' at age 19. Now aged 20, she is hoping to return to college as an adult to study A level music. Thereafter she hopes to study composition – and further confront and overcome her problems with musical theory and notation.

Annemarie Sand was born in Denmark and came to England to study at the Royal Academy of Music and the London Opera Studio. She made her professional opera debut at English National Opera. She has performed throughout Europe in major opera, oratorio and concert roles, and has appeared for the BBC as both soloist in promenade concerts and as singer on the sound track for a TV series. Her repertoire is wide and covers both traditional and contemporary roles. A highlight of her 2000 season was her singing of the critical role of Sieglinde in Wagner's *Die Walküre*.

Olly Smith is currently finishing his undergraduate music degree at the University of Wales, Bangor. After graduation and further training he hopes to pursue a career as a music teacher and performer on the recorder.

John Westcombe was originally a teacher; thereafter he held senior adviser/inspector posts in three large local educational authorities. He led successful teaching teams in both curriculum and performance areas and directed concerts in national venues both in Britain and abroad. Recent work includes evaluating music education projects for national bodies, co-leading teachers' and sixth formers' courses, and writing. His *Careers in Music* is published by Heinemann. He has a close association with Broxbourne Dyslexia Unit.

Jacob Wiltshire was diagnosed as severely dyslexic at the age of 7. He attended a school with a specialist dyslexia unit until the age of 11. Now aged 17, Jacob is studying music technology and sound engineering. He plays guitar and percussion by ear, while also composing electronic music using a computer-sequencing program. He recently gained nine GCSEs between grades A and C, including a B in Music.

Siw Wood reports that 'dyslexia has had a huge influence on my life', and that she was 'considered too hopeless at spelling' to go to secretarial college. She did, in fact, go to art college but never used her art to earn money until she came to live in Wales ten years ago. Her jobs have included dental nurse, laboratory assistant, ward orderly in a mental hospital, farm worker, seller of merchandise, public relations official in a theatre, disabled persons' mobility assistant, and chauffeur. Her main hobby is singing.

Foreword

Now that dyslexia is an acknowledged syndrome, not a condition invented by the middle classes to excuse the academic non-success of some of their children (and it was so regarded by the Department of Education 20 years ago, indeed probably more recently), it is well recognized that dyslexic people, children and adults, have specific difficulties with reading, spelling and writing, and probably with number. What this excellent collection of essays reminds us is that dyslexia also manifests itself in difficulties with concentration, with short-term memory, with coordination, and with the organization of work. These difficulties may be just as crippling and frustrating as those that are more widely recognized.

People who have a deep feeling for music and perhaps a fine and accurate ear for it may therefore be frustrated not only by the problem of learning musical notation but by the difficulties of coordinating eye and hand, of following instructions or of looking from their written page or score to the conductor without losing their place in the score. Above all, dyslexic people need more time to bring their activities together than the dynamic of music allows them. Music, as one of them says, does not allow stops – or not at the point where the performer may need to stop.

The optimistic message of all the fascinating and often moving contributions that the editors have brought together is that people who love music and are determined can find strategies to overcome almost all their difficulties, and that, in doing so, they also increase their general competence. One of the most moving stories is of the little girl who dismally failed her pre-grade 1 piano examination because, stumbling upstairs to the appointed room, she was so much disorientated that she fell off the piano stool and ended up at the wrong part of the keyboard – and could not find middle C. Yet she passed with distinction next time round. Such courage is remarkable and the boost to her confidence in the end must have been beyond everything.

Just as remarkable is the evidence, from a wide-ranging enquiry, of the way in which dyslexic choristers learn to succeed. Here the confidence they gain from being accepted as choristers on the basis of their talent is equalled only by what they gain from the discipline of the choir and of the music itself, and the camaraderie with their fellow choristers. This shows, I think, that despite the relentless pressures to which they are subjected they are helped in every aspect of their lives by their own growing professionalism and the strategies they have, perforce, to adopt to overcome their natural lack of organization.

I hope this book will be widely read by anyone, parent, teacher or employer, who may have contact with dyslexia. It is a tribute to the courage and determination of musicians; but it is also eye-opening about what it is actually like to be dyslexic. The editors as well as the contributors are to be congratulated.

Baroness Warnock
President, British Dyslexia Association

Preface

This book draws on the experiences of a number of individuals who share a common interest in music and dyslexia. The contributors include teachers in most sectors of music education and both professional and amateur musicians. Some of them are themselves dyslexic or have dyslexic relatives and can therefore speak of dyslexia at first hand. There is a wide span of ages. Many of those who have contributed are members of the Music Committee of the British Dyslexia Association (BDA).

The earliest meetings of this group date back to the 1980s. The initiator was Pam Smith who at the time was working for the Disabled Living Foundation. It was Pam who, at the instigation of Daphne Kennard, called us together in the first place, and it was also she who with the group's help was responsible for editing the first BDA booklet on music and dyslexia. The other members of the group were Margaret Hubicki, Violet Brand, Janet Coker, Caroline Beaumont (afterwards Caroline Symes), and Tim Miles. For various reasons the Disabled Living Foundation was unable to continue supporting our work, but fortunately the BDA undertook to provide the necessary financial backing to keep the group in existence. From these earliest beginnings we have grown into a committee of 11 members who meet regularly about four or five times a year.

People sometimes raise the question 'Can music be a *cure* for dyslexia?' From the point of view of this book such a question represents a misunderstanding. As will be made plain in a number of the chapters, being dyslexic has both advantages and disadvantages – and no one would wish to 'cure' the advantages! With regard to the disadvantages, rather than speaking of 'curing' them it is perhaps more appropriate to think in terms of providing dyslexic individuals with appropriate strategies so that the possible adverse effects of their dyslexia can be minimized. It is possible that musical activity may assist other sectors of learning, for instance the singing of traditional action songs (compare Overy, 2000). However, 'music therapy' – in the sense of using music to remove people's stresses and tensions – is an entirely different matter and is outside the scope of this book.

Some ideas may occur in the book more than once. The editors have knowingly left these in place since they serve to underline the fact that certain strategies have seemed important to more than one contributor. The book is first and foremost a record of people's experiences, and these may or may not be similar.

None of the chapters except Chapters 5 and 11 has appeared previously in its present form. In the case of Chapter 5, contributed by Caroline Oldfield, we wish to thank the editors of *Pan* magazine, the Journal of the British Flute Society, for permission to reprint this material. In the case of Chapter 11, contributed by Jacob Wiltshire, thanks are due to John Wiley & Sons, publishers of *Dyslexia: An International Journal of Research and Practice Volume 2(1)*, where Jacob's paper first appeared.

The materials described in Chapter 20 (Margaret Hubicki's 'Colour-Staff') appeared commercially in the 1970s but the chapter in its existing form is new.

While gathering these different contributions we have encountered several 'gems' which we wanted to share with our readers. That on p. 17 will already be well known to dyslexia specialists, but is nevertheless worth repeating. These 'gems' have been placed in 'boxes' at the end of some of the chapters. The chapter's author is not responsible for them except in the case of those at the end of chapters 4, 6 and 9.

The book is not concerned with dyslexics' spelling, so all spelling errors have been corrected. The only exception to this principle will be found in Chapter 17, where the misspellings of James, the chorister described by Sheila Oglethorpe, have been retained because they illustrate how a successful chorister may still have to struggle in this area.

At the end of the book we have included some suggestions for further reading. These are followed by the reference section, which documents all the references that have appeared in the previous chapters.

We have taken 'Opening new doors' as our subtitle. It is our hope that if all the relevant agencies – parents, schools, colleges, friends, councils, teachers and music tutors, to name only a few – use their best endeavours, these doors will be found to be at least partially open.

Finally, we should like to express our gratitude to the British Dyslexia Association for the support given to the Music and Dyslexia committee over the years, and to Joanne Rule in particular for her active and positive encouragement.

TR Miles and John Westcombe
November 2000

Chapter 1
The manifestations of dyslexia, its biological bases, and its effects on daily living

TR MILES

The manifestations of dyslexia

Those who have worked with dyslexic children or adults are frequently left with a sense of incongruity – with the impression that there is something that does not 'add up'. What one regularly notices is the *unevenness* of their performance: one is tempted to ask how it is that most dyslexics find a particular task so difficult whereas most non-dyslexics find it so easy, and, conversely, how some other seemingly difficult tasks cause dyslexics no problems at all.

As is well known, one of the most noticeable ways in which this incongruity shows itself, at least as far as the English language is concerned, is in the area of literacy. Most dyslexics, although they eventually learn to read, are late in doing so, and even in adulthood most of them are still relatively poor spellers. Even when they have learned to read they usually remain slow readers, and some of them report that they avoid reading unless it is really necessary.

There is in dyslexia an underlying pattern that is easy to recognize once one has seen a small number of cases. Dyslexia is sometimes described as a *syndrome* (Critchley, 1981; Galaburda, 1999); this implies a cluster or group of manifest-ations that form a meaningful whole despite a wide range of individual differences. Information on what to look for if you suspect that a child is dyslexic will be found in Appendix I, along with a list of *dos* and *dont's* that have been found useful over the years. Pointers to dyslexia in adults will be found in Appendix II.

Besides literacy difficulties, one of the most common manifestations, both in children and in adults, is a poor short-term memory. For example, many dyslexics find it difficult to memorize a series of instructions or a sequence of names such as the months of the year, and many of them have difficulty in learning 'times tables' in arithmetic (Miles, 1993). Dyslexics vary in intelligence as much as non-dyslexics, but because some items in traditional intelligence tests are affected by their dyslexia, for example their ability to recall a series of digits or to carry out at speed

1

calculations requiring a knowledge of 'times tables', it is hazardous, to say the least, to try to assign precise IQ figures (Miles, 1996).

As dyslexic tendencies can sometimes be passed via the genes, it is important to check whether anyone else in the family has similar strengths and weaknesses. If the answer to this is 'no', it is still possible that manifestations of dyslexia will be present in a particular individual. However, if several members of the family are known to be affected it is very likely indeed that there will be dyslexic manifest-ations in one or more of their relatives, even though there may be considerable variety in the extent to which they are inconvenienced or handicapped. Dyslexia is in fact more common in males than in females, probably by a ratio of about 4:1 (Miles, Haslum, and Wheeler, 1998), although the reason for this is still a matter of speculation.

It will be seen from the two appendixes that the criteria for dyslexia vary at different ages in childhood and are different again in the case of adults. If a 5-year-old puts figures the wrong way round, writes 'b' for 'd', or has not learned how to use the labels 'left' and 'right', one should not immediately conclude that the child is dyslexic. What one needs to look out for is the persistence of difficulties when other children have grown out of them.

In the case of a young child, if there is any doubt about a diagnosis of dyslexia it is crucial to err on the side of caution; this means assuming that the child *will* have problems with reading and spelling, and it means taking immediate steps to provide the appropriate teaching. If the difficulties are not as severe as one feared, this is a bonus, and the special teaching will have done no harm. In contrast, what is called the 'false negative' – that is, saying that children are not dyslexic when in fact they are – can lead to years of frustration and increasing loss of confidence.

In the case of both children and adults it is important to take account of the whole picture. Anyone on a particular occasion may muddle up 'left' and 'right' without this being evidence for dyslexia; but if individuals persistently do so – and in addition are poor spellers, cannot learn their 'times tables' despite ample oppor-tunity, and have uncles who, despite adequate intelligence, were reluctant ever to open a book, the accumulation of signs, rather than any one sign on its own, adds up to dyslexia.

The necessary special arrangements in terms of extra teaching help, extra time in examinations, and so forth, if a person is found to be dyslexic will vary from one individual to another. Their needs will, of course, be different at different ages. One of the main functions of the word 'dyslexia' is to force people to ask themselves whether these needs are being properly met. In the case of any disability, if one does not describe it in terms of a recognized label it is only by the merest accident that one will end up doing the right thing.

A central message for readers of this book is that there are few things that are *totally impossible* for dyslexics if they are sufficiently determined and are given (or discover for themselves) the appropriate compensatory strategies. It is possible that, because of an inherent physiological limitation, it is difficult for dyslexics to deal with symbolic information that is presented at speed (see below), but how much 'speeding up' is possible is not yet known.

The biological bases of dyslexia

For practising teachers a detailed knowledge of the biological bases of dyslexia is unnecessary. Those wishing for a brief summary of some of the main points in the evidence should consult Miles and Miles (1999, Chapters 7, 8 and 9). More technical information will be found in a number of different sources, for instance Pennington (1991), Reid Lyon and Rumsey (1996), and Nicolson et al. (1999). Pennington's book deals with genetic and neurological influences on dyslexia; that by Reid Lyon and Rumsey provides information about brain-scanning techniques – MRI (magnetic resonance imaging) and PET (positron emission tomography) – while the paper by Nicolson et al. provides evidence that dyslexics display minor malfunctioning of the cerebellum.

From the 1980s onwards the area of the brain chosen for special investigation by dyslexia researchers was the *planum temporale* – a region on the upper surface of the temporal lobe on either side of the brain. Earlier autopsy studies had shown that in about 65% to 75% of unselected brains the two plana were asymmetrical and of different sizes, the planum on the left side usually being the larger. In a study of the brains of eight individuals known to have been dyslexic in their lifetime it was found that in all eight cases the two plana were symmetrical.

A further finding from the autopsy studies was that the brains of the dyslexics contained an abnormal number of malformations, known as *ectopias*. These are believed to have arisen because the migration of cells to the cerebral cortex, which takes place in the months before birth, was incomplete, with the consequence that the cells ended up out of place.

It has also been shown that within the visual system of humans and other primates it is possible to distinguish two separate pathways that contain different types of cell – large cells that respond to fast-moving, low-contrast information (the *magnocellular* pathway), and smaller cells that respond to slow-moving high-contrast information (the *parvocellular* pathway). When five of the eight dyslexic brains were re-examined it was found that there was nothing unusual about the parvocellular pathways but that there were abnormalities of the magnocellular pathway – the cell bodies were smaller and more variable in size and shape (Livingstone et al., 1991). It seems likely that there are similar magnocellular abnormalities in the auditory system (Galaburda and Livingstone, 1993).

What, then, is the significance of all these findings for the practising teacher?

The first point of importance is the recognition that the difficulties experienced by dyslexics do, indeed, have a biological basis; in other words they arise as a direct result of the individual's constitutional make-up. This represents a change from what was commonly believed by educationalists until about the 1960s. Before this time, if a child had difficulty in learning to read and spell it was widely assumed that the causes were solely environmental. For example it might be suggested that the teaching was poor, or that the parents were over fussy and created so much pressure that their children reacted against this by refusing to learn. When one looks back one is forced to say that some of these explanations seem to have been based on the most slender evidence. The central difficulty, however, is that explanations in terms of 'family dynamics' put the cart before the horse!

A dyslexic child may indeed feel under pressure, and, in the absence of sympathetic handling, may indeed become discouraged and stop trying to learn. Once it is recognized, however, that the original cause of the child's literacy problems is constitutional the situation needs to be seen in a new light. *Of course* a child with a constitutionally caused limitation may feel discouraged – and may stop trying on the grounds that this is preferable to trying and failing. *Of course* parents may feel worried about their child's lack of progress. These, however, are the consequences, not the causes, of the child's literacy difficulties, and are quite understandable as a reaction to them. It also follows that neither the child nor the parents need blame themselves for the difficulties – any more than anyone is to be blamed if a child turns out to be colour-blind. On this different view of the situation, if a dyslexic child is struggling or misbehaving there is the opportunity for the teacher to show understanding ('no wonder you felt discouraged') and to be positive and praise effort rather than blame the child for not 'trying harder'.

The fact that ectopias are associated with dyslexia and can be detected before birth suggests that, whatever the later environmental influences, there is *in utero* the potentiality for being dyslexic. Thus although the right kind of teaching can minimize the disadvantages of being dyslexic, it is no longer possible to believe that poor teaching on its own is sufficient to cause the problems.

The fact that there may be a mild cerebellar deficiency makes sense of the familiar observation that some dyslexics are clumsy and poorly co-ordinated and some have very untidy handwriting. It is possible (although this is more speculative) that the poor sense of rhythm shown by some otherwise musically gifted dyslexics is also cerebellar in origin.

It has also been suggested that the so-called 'phonological' difficulties shown by dyslexics – that is, their difficulties with the memorization and ordering of speech sounds – are caused by faults in the auditory magnocellular system. It is possible that if sounds are presented in very rapid succession the dyslexic brain is relatively inefficient at dealing with them. However, one should remember that, as far as we know, playing notes at speed is not as such a problem for dyslexics, and one must therefore suppose that their limitation affects them not in muscular movement as such but only when material has to be named.

Finally, it has been suggested that there is significance in the fact that in the dyslexic brains examined to date the two plana were symmetrical. This well-established fact has unfortunately led to some rather wild speculation. There is firm evidence that in most individuals it is the left half of the brain that controls speech, and it is likely, although not certain, that it is the right half that makes possible the recognition of patterns and the ability to view things as 'wholes'. It therefore makes sense to suppose that in the case of dyslexics it is the left hemisphere that is relatively weak and the right hemisphere that is relatively strong. If this is correct it would also make sense of the familiar observation that it is the *balance* of skills in dyslexics that is unusual: they are relatively weak at what are apparently 'left hemisphere' tasks – reading, spelling, and the memorization of symbolic material – and relatively strong at apparently 'right hemisphere' tasks, for instance those required for success in art, architecture, and engineering.

Building on this idea, West (1997) has presented a series of biographical sketches that suggest that there have been some individuals – his examples include Michael Faraday, Thomas Alva Edison, and William Butler Yeats – who were creative precisely because of this unusual balance of skills. On West's view the demand for those with dyslexic tendencies may well increase in the near future, particularly now that much of the 'clerical' work (accurate copying, punctuating, adding up columns of figures, and so forth) can be carried out by computer. The fact that there are 'positive' aspects to dyslexia is a theme that will be recurring throughout this book.

I end this section with a few speculations on musical ability. It is possible, although by no means certain, that appreciation of music is largely a function of the right hemisphere. If this is so it becomes particularly important to distinguish between the *sounds* of music and *musical notation* (compare Hubicki and Miles, 1991). We would not normally expect dyslexics to be good at sight-reading, because this involves rapid translation of marks on paper into muscular movements; nor in view of their memory problems would we expect them to be good at memorizing the individual notes of a piece of music. They may, indeed, *end up* by being at least as successful as their non-dyslexic colleagues, but one's impression is that success is achieved only after very hard work and the use of suitable compensatory strategies. In contrast, we would not be at all surprised if some of them showed extreme musical sensitivity, including awareness of the music as a whole. The evidence in the chapters that follow suggests that this may well be the case.

The effects of dyslexia in daily living

Where there is an understanding of dyslexia in both the home and the school its adverse effects can be minimized. In an unsympathetic environment, however, all sorts of things can go wrong. Thus if a teacher returns a child's written work with a mass of spelling corrections – possibly in red ink, to make things worse! – and writes such things as, '2 out of 10; take more trouble with your spelling' but gives no indication as to how the spelling might be improved, such a teacher would do well to reflect on what he or she is *doing* to that child and what is its effect on that child's self-esteem. It is particularly galling if the child has in fact spent many hours on the task and, because there is little to show for it, is then scolded for lack of effort.

If a dyslexic child misremembers a message – as often happens because of their limitations in short-term memory – a parent or teacher unaware of the complications caused by dyslexia may say unsympathetically, 'Why didn't you listen?' Similarly, children with a poor sense of time who fail to turn up for an appointment or have forgotten to bring their gym shoes ('didn't you *know* it was Wednesday?') are that much more vulnerable than their classmates and more liable to be 'picked on' by an unsympathetic teacher. If these were once-off events they might not have any lasting effect, but if they happen week after week and year after year throughout both primary and secondary education it is scarcely surprising that some dyslexics feel very unsure of themselves.

The social difficulties of the dyslexic do not always go away in adulthood. In general there is the perpetual worry that one may have 'got it wrong'. The following examples are drawn from my own experience.

A successful dyslexic businessman could read more or less adequately if he did not feel under pressure, but if a subordinate handed him a balance sheet with the question 'What do you think of this?' his usual policy was to 'stall' by saying 'I will take it home and look at it later.' This normally worked satisfactorily. However, at one point in his life he had been appointed to the office of 'Chairman of the Guild' – a prestigious honour given in recognition of his services to industry. Out of the blue, at the time of the ceremony, he suddenly heard the (for him) awesome words, 'I call on our new chairman to read the rules of the Guild.' In the stress of that particular moment there was no way in which he could have read anything aloud without stumblings and hesitations. He was reduced to saying that he was unwell and to retreating unceremoniously from the room.

In another case a dyslexic adult who worked for a law firm had been accused of falsifying the records. When I questioned him about this charge he said, 'Someone got me to sign papers . . . I filled in three forms with long chassis numbers (20 figures) – these had come in the wrong position . . . I have difficulty in reading . . . lengthy legal documents. You pretend you have read it so as not to hold up a meeting.' He also mentioned the difficulties that he had when he was in a bank or had to sign his name when the shop assistant was watching.

Not long ago, at Crewe station, a dyslexic adult was looking for platform '9' where she had been told that there was a train to Bangor. She misread '9' for '6' and discovered her mistake only when the train at platform '6' was just about to leave for Glasgow! Two dyslexic teenagers were looking for Kensington, but having misread the signs on the underground found themselves alighting at Kennington. It is of course true that such mistakes are not limited to dyslexics, but one's impression is that dyslexics are more vulnerable.

Sometimes the disadvantages may seem trivial but they can still be very humiliating to a sensitive dyslexic. For example, one adult reported to me that he had had to stop playing darts because of his slowness in calculating the number required for the next throw; he explained that keeping the other players waiting had become too much of an embarrassment.

It is not surprising when such things happen that they affect the dyslexics self-esteem. The following is an account by my colleague, Dorothy Gilroy, of her experiences with students who despite their dyslexia had been successful in getting to university.

> The students I have worked with quite often compare themselves unfavourably with their peer group. In listening to a spontaneous, undirected general conversation lasting about 20 minutes between five students, the following words and phrases were noted: 'hopeless at' (seven times); 'useless at' (five times); 'could never' (three times); 'mess' (twice); 'typical me' (twice); 'never been any good at' . . . It seems that, as a result of a lifetime of mishaps, some dyslexics adults consistently undervalue themselves. (Gilroy, 1995: 66–7)

Similar low self-esteem has also been reported by Riddick et al. (1999).

The lesson to be learned from these and other examples is that dyslexia does not leave you and may show its effects when you are least expecting them. However, now that there is increasing awareness of dyslexia among the public at large one may hope that the pressure on dyslexics to 'cover up' their difficulties will become very much less.

Chapter 2
How dyslexia can affect musicians

JOHN WESTCOMBE

The following conversation took place some years ago at a youth orchestra audition: smartly presented trombonist says 'I am going to play *Sophisticated Lady* by Ben Elton.' Music adviser suggests that perhaps the candidate has the composer wrong. Candidate looks in music and says 'Sorry, I am going to play *Sophisticated Lady* by Elton John'. Music adviser, seeing embarrassment arising, asks whether it could . . . er . . . possibly be by Duke Ellington. Candidate looks in his music again and says, in a perfect put-down, 'If you knew that in the first place why didn't you tell me?' I was the music adviser involved and, regrettably, only some months after did I realize that the lad probably had dyslexic traits, was reading inaccurately, and had mixed up the order of his 'ell's and 'ton's. After his audition we invited him to join the orchestra.

Many of us have been close to a similar situation, where assumptions are made, for example about the ability of a good piano player to sight-read something at a choir rehearsal, and it has been necessary for someone to explain that that is just what the player does not want – to be shown up by failing.

There have been many encouraging developments recently in the field of dyslexia. In particular there has been research into brain function and genetics, with consequent acceptance by the scientific community of the existence of dyslexia as a clinical condition, and people have come to recognize its effects on musicians. On the musical side, a sizeable number of books and articles have been written (for details see the references section), courses for teachers have been organized, especially by Violet Brand and Margaret Hubicki, and in suitable cases special arrangements for dyslexic candidates in both grade examinations and public examinations in school are made by examination boards. In the wider area of learning difficulties there have been a number of claims made by parents against Local Education Authorities (LEAs) for lack of early diagnosis and there has been concern at failure in some initial teacher training courses to make prospective teachers aware of the dyslexic's problems. Happily, some more systematic training has latterly been developed for existing teachers in some LEAs. Other relevant facts have also come to light, not least the probable existence in some dyslexics of superior three-dimensional skills, some of which are needed in architecture, and the ability of internationally known people to succeed in their careers despite the initial handicaps of dyslexia.

It has been pleasing to those of us who have tutored on this subject to the Associated Board of the Royal Schools of Music (ABRSM) teachers' certificate groups that, each year, a greater number of course members have taught music pupils with dyslexic traits and have already modified their approaches and techniques.

It is the experience of many of us that dyslexics can sometimes be extremely creative, for example by coming up with new and original solutions to mathematical problems or by noticing patterns and relationships that their non-dyslexic peers may sometimes miss. Whether these abilities are the consequence of a different brain organization is not yet confirmed. What seems clear from experience is that some of them can show extreme musical sensitivity. One has the impression, too, that for some people the reading of music is easier than the reading of words and that for others it is the other way round. Whether this is due to some inherent properties of musical and alphabetic notation, however, or whether it is the result of effort and interest is not clear.

Dyslexia has no correlation with intelligence. The result of this on the musical side is that there are many examples of very bright young musicians being extremely frustrated by its effects. Thus there may be difficulties in singing back any but the shortest of musical phrases, and some dyslexics have difficulty in recalling the notes in the right order. This last is unlikely when only two or three notes have to be memorized, but it has been known for a player to deliver a whole line of music backwards!

There is sometimes difficulty in arranging items in sequence (for example, the letters of the alphabet or the months of the year), and in the world of music this may show itself as a difficulty experienced when they are asked to play something back or in getting to rota-based instrumental lessons on time. Teachers need to be aware of this and also to know that there is a strong pull for a musician with dyslexic traits to want to go back to the beginning of a piece rather than work on a tricky short passage, which in any case they find difficult to relocate in the score. In fact, general organizational skills (bringing lunch and the right music) will often not come easily, and if some of the above trials appear in combination we begin to understand the agonies and feelings of failure that arise. In the telling words of one music student, the situation is 'like getting down on your starting blocks for the 100 metres and finding it's the 110 metres high hurdles'. However, with care and patience the appropriate skills can be learned. In particular, many of those dyslexics who are approaching critical public examinations such as General Certificate of Secondary Education (GCSE), Advanced ('A') Level, or Grade VIII have often been found to succeed in bringing order at least to timing and concentration in their general lives – and in obtaining high grades.

Early diagnosis is essential, and patient support and understanding can reduce some of the basic problems before the need arises for the decoding of musical notation. Patience may also be required when pupils seem to need a long pause before starting to play, or when they are camouflaging their lack of reading powers by trying to learn a piece from memory. However, some traits do not disappear, and mature musicians can sometimes continue to be affected by their relative lack of skill at sight reading. One dyslexic musician has described the situation as follows:

> The notes take longer to absorb and are less easy to retrieve . . . I just need more time to process the symbols. I think I'm less organized than my friends, am no good with maps, but feel very creative in the parts of my music-making which do not depend on notation. As a singer, I need my accompanist to play my line repeatedly, but once I have really slogged away at it, and put some of my own bold markings on the music to denote key and mood changes etc., I'm all right. Otherwise, it could feel like sight-reading every time I looked at it.

It has been salutary to hear that some musicians have proceeded through training to earning a living *without knowing* that they had problems in the reading of music! Put another way, the above quote explains that initial memorizing is difficult and the usual processes cannot all be brought to bear at the same time when the musician wants them. It is possible for a dyslexic musician to work hard to play a short extract accurately without realizing that it constitutes a known tune. It seems that non-dyslexics are unaware of this problem.

Not all dyslexics can recognize that when two words end with the same combination of letters, such as *yield* and *field,* that these words *rhyme.* This has great import musically as things happen in music that are analogous to the rhyming of words. For example the composer brings the phrase to a close, or uses a short rhythmic fragment to highlight the nature of the closing 'syllables'. Similarly dyslexics may find dance steps hard to remember – of interest to those teachers working with both beginners and advanced pupils integrating music and all aspects of movement.

For some children there are problems over the words 'high' and 'low': one only has to watch an infants' class stretching 'up and down' to the teacher's instructions and one will find that two or three of them will always be watching the others and copying them. Nor will a dyslexic child necessarily appreciate that notes played on the piano by the left hand will normally be lower in pitch that notes played by the right hand. There are many professional musicians who have recognized that without systematic teaching of such things – and going over them many times – they would have given up long ago. Teachers need to know that expected connections may not be made or implications understood. There is a telling story of a youngster appearing to make no progress until it was realized that the note she was intending to play was the one coinciding with 'the other end of the stalk', not where, for example, the crotchet or quaver was shown!

Decoding and music's own inconsistencies

The main challenge of musical notation is that of decoding: one is learning a new language, just as one would be in the case of Sanskrit. Those who read musical notation have to deal with an additional set of symbols – when even familiar alphabetic symbols are difficult for them. More speculatively, it has been suggested that notation sometimes appears to fall away from the horizontal or seems watery. Whether or not this often happens, there can be no doubt that in the reading of music, just as in the reading of print, the eye likes to move on ahead, and a dyslexic who cannot do this easily is likely to find sight-reading difficult.

Musical notation contains a number of characteristics that are potentially puzzling. The time signatures are not fractions; notes that have to be played on a horizontal keyboard are written vertically on the stave; our hands on the piano keyboard are mirror images of each other, with the result that the thumb of the left hand normally plays the highest note in the bass clef while the thumb of the right hand normally plays the lowest note of the treble clef. A non-dyslexic musician may either not notice such things or not be troubled by them; the dyslexic musician, however, is more vulnerable and cannot always make the necessary adjustments. This is chiefly because there is a large amount of information on the printed page – information that indicates what notes to play, how to play them (loudly, softly, with feeling, and so forth), and when to deliver them – either on one's own or simultaneously with others. Nor should we forget the added complications that there are occasions, particularly for percussionists, when a large number of empty bars have to be accurately counted. An extra challenge is that directions as to style of playing are often given in an unfamiliar language, viz. by means of foreign words such as *adagio, andante, lentement*.

Thus to ensure that the correct notes are played at the correct time there needs to be co-ordination of the inputs from the eye, the ear, and the muscles in the hand. Two of the main difficulties for the dyslexic are slowness in processing symbolic information (Miles, 1993: 136) and delay in acquiring automaticity (Nicolson et al., 1999). For all these reasons, reading music from a score creates many kinds of difficulty for the dyslexic.

Moreover a musician in an orchestra has to follow and interpret many different actions and gestures. There are also problems of organization. Thus to a percussion player moving around between four instruments and music sheets on three different stands, the conductor saying 'Right folks, 23 bars before letter H' is not good news. Finding letter H in the score is bad enough, and counting 23 bars provides many opportunities for error. Just as having to look up and down from the board to the teacher raises problems for the dyslexic in the classroom, so there are problems in an orchestra when dyslexic players need to switch their visual attention from the conductor to their music stand to their instrument and back again while sustaining their aural concentration.

There are further paradoxes in musical notation. Thus a fingering chart for the flute that shows the flute vertically may be confusing to a dyslexic flute player. Half the string instruments in an orchestra ('cellos and basses) produce higher notes as the left hand moves away from the body, while for the remainder the reverse is the case. The bassoon has a downwards-then-upwards fingering sequence whereas the sound continues to go down. Also while the hands on most instruments are fingering or holding, those on the harp are largely 'off' the instrument, and the pedal changes must be made strictly in sequence. However we know of dyslexic harpists who have been successfully brought through those problems. Interestingly, a brass tutor working in a special school has had success teaching the cornet by putting valve numbers under the music (not always thought good practice). When questioned about brass instruments' properties of producing different notes with the same fingering through changing lip pressure, he said 'Ah, that's where their listening powers come in but I do have to play it through for them first.'

Conversely, training in choirs involving the artificial separation of syllables, pronunciation of foreign languages and emphasizing of critical consonants seems very beneficial, even though there is the added factor of having to deliver both words and musical line (see Chapter 17).

It has been pointed out that when skilled readers read newspapers and book material they scan for gist rather than attending to each letter or word separately. In music, however, accuracy is essential. In much of the music repertoire people can tell at once when notes are wrong, and a rough guess at what the chord ought to be just will not do. However, the notion of general contour (or sense of direction) is helpful in all stages of music learning, and some professional musicians who have dyslexic traits find a 'grand audio plan' of a song or piece helps to hold things together (see Chapter 6).

Some of what is outlined above has emerged through the concentrated exchanges possible in very small groups or one-to-one discussion, or through assessment procedures sought by a parent highlighting something not previously perceived. In schools there are class, instrumental and vocal teachers who wax eloquent about there being no time to deal with pupils individually when most of their day is with medium or large groups. It will be the case, though, that other agencies in the school will also know of the pupil's needs, and joint approaches help to share the responsibility. Also a brief word of praise to a pupil for hard work on a task goes a long way!

I have exposed the difficulties of the dyslexic at some length because, as teachers, parents and friends, we need to understand as much as possible about the musical manifestations of dyslexia and to be aware of the clues for which we should look. Indeed it is a fascinating detective matter. Fortunately, we have come a long way from the days when it was said that dyslexia was an excuse made by middle-class parents of children who were in fact slow learners. The evidence that this is not so seems decisive (Miles, Wheeler, and Haslum, 1994). The latest medical research based on magnetic resonance imaging (MRI) is enormously exciting, and if we also take into account the well-established finding that dyslexia is sometimes inherited (see Chapter 1) it seems likely that there are good prospects of growth across the whole area. I would suggest that if a clearer view of tracking between the decoding and sense-and-understanding areas can be gained it will have great import for music.

Strategies for teaching

How, then, can we best help dyslexic musicians? Most teaching strategies apply both in class and in one-to-one situations. It is, of course, important to understand that teaching needs differ from one individual to another, as is made plain in many other chapters of this book.

Advice includes:

- Be on the lookout for the signs described above and for those mentioned in the appendixes. Make sure that someone has checked that other possible causes of the difficulties, such as uncorrected eyesight or of hearing problems, have been excluded.
- In explaining the difficulties to parents, teachers, and the children themselves be as explicit as possible and make clear that nothing is being held back.
- Be lenient towards people who lose their place in the music. Ringing the first note of important phrases gives an alternative reference point, thus obviating the need to go back to the beginning.
- Bear in mind that some dyslexics may use memorization as a way of compensation for their poor reading – and may not do so accurately. Remember that children may not be genuinely reading when you think they are – it may be a form of camouflage! Such camouflage is particularly likely to occur in the early weeks of learning a new piece and may indicate that they are trying to defeat the 'looks like sight-reading every time I return to it' problem.
- Provide plenty of opportunities to revise previous work.
- Play music to them regularly. This is analogous to reading stories aloud: in both cases one is giving the pupils something that they can enjoy without too much expenditure of effort. When playing with them sometimes stand alongside them, not always opposite them.
- Emphasize the need for them to look carefully, to listen carefully, and to be consciously aware of their hand movements. As in the case of literacy, the teaching needs to be multisensory.
- There may be pupils who are puzzled by the fact that the names of the notes run from A to G and no further. Some of them may appreciate the beautiful physical symmetry that this notation implies. For example, one note, 'A' sounds at 220 cycles per second (cps) and the next one up sounds at precisely twice that

number of cps. If one called the notes 'H', 'I', 'J', 'K', etc. this symmetry would be lost (see also Chapter 20).

- In class the glockenspiel can be turned by 90 degrees (marching bands have it on a pole) so that what is *heard* as high or low is also *seen* as high or low. Similarly, enlarged music can be written so as to line up with the keys on a piano.
- A useful mnemonic is that the abbreviation *dim*. (*diminuendo* – becoming softer) can be associated with dimming the lights.
- Explain the inconsistency of stave-letters (in particular EBGDF on the treble stave and GBDFA on the bass) by inserting middle C between the two. This has the effect of temporarily closing up the two staves. Middle C has exactly this central position on the 11-line great staff – a device sometimes used to fix clefs. Thus the two familiar clefs, bass and treble, are a continuous sequence but have the ability to extend towards each other, allowing middle C to be available both above the one and below the other (see also Chapter 20).
- Keep your mnemonics for remembering the letter names up to date. For example a pupil interested in football might be told, in the vernacular of ex-England soccer coaches, **E**xcellent **G**ame **B**eckham **D**one **F**abulous.
- Some people with dyslexic traits find placing a coloured transparency over the music helps. There appear to be individual differences as regards the most suitable colour (see Miles and Miles, 1999: Chapter 7).
- Some pupils may find a single-line instrument a better starting point than the piano.
- Some musicians do not like words written on the music, but cues and reminders can sometimes be helpful. For example, it may be useful to highlight patterns that have appeared previously, or to increase the size of small signs such as the repeat colon .
- In the early stages attaching a non-musical association to a technical fact sometimes helps. For example, the pupil can think of A major with three sharps as the three bears/wise men/musketeers scale (even though the examiner is not going to call it by any of these names).
- Say 'Play it with this/that hand' not 'Play it with the left/right hand'. Do not say 'Where were we?' but 'How's that minuet coming on?'
- Try not to overload the pupil with information and give the information time to 'sink in'. To say 'Watch the octave key in bar eight during the diminuendo' makes too many demands all at once.

Further thoughts

Even when they have received no adequate diagnosis many musicians with dyslexia have struggled on, having in the first place brought their own clever strategies to bear on their problems and later with the help of sensitive and above all systematic teaching. Some of the stories are very moving. In particular, one of the biggest challenges is that of coping with the feeling that you ought to be able to do a task but finding yourself frustrated by something that you do not understand. The ways in which many musical dyslexics have responded to this are truly striking, and their determination is heroic!

Since sight-reading is one of the most awkward of decoding problems, the ability to overcome feelings of panic may come only gradually. Examining Boards rightly insist that there should be no dilution of standards in the case of dyslexic candidates, but have ruled that in the case of sight-reading they may have extra time in which to look at the piece to be played.

While seeking to help a guitarist recently, I discovered that although he had written markings, for example 'F ma' at the beginning of a bar, it had not occurred to him that in a sight-reading situation at least some of the melody in that bar might be the notes of the scale of F. From another angle, a string player may say 'this' (a finger placement) 'is E' more readily than 'the third space of the stave is E'.

Dyslexics sometimes feel that they are the victims of discrimination. On this, the Director of the Royal Opera House chorus made the helpful point that a dyslexic singer (all other things being equal) would neither be turned down nor be uncomfortable with them because the chorus rehearsals may span many months. There was a possible difficulty, however, for those entering the field of recording sessions. Here versatility was at a premium since virtually everything was sight read on the day and could be in any of five languages.

Some reminders

We already know that singing can help non-dyslexics to learn the alphabet and arithmetical tables, and it is seems true in general that the *rhythms* of music can aid memorization. We need to find the ways in which each individual pupil makes most progress, teach to their strengths, and encourage them to analyse their own learning style. This of course should be true of all teaching, although in practice, sadly, this is not always the case.

Notation should be seen for what it is – there are plenty of ways of making music without it. Thus we can enjoy listening to it; and we can play sounds from other cultures where notation is not used. We can improvise in the classroom, in the jazz club and in the cathedral organ loft. As a result of play-and-print technology we can even compose it without ourselves having to write the traditional notation by hand. As one individual said, 'Reading music is hard; making it up and listening closely is easy'.

While hoping that the pupil reflects on his or her mode of learning, we need to adjust. It may be important that we get the pupil to reflect on and analyse his or her learning style, but, equally, that we adjust our teaching styles and parental support to the needs of the pupil. It is these two in conjunction that may unlock a door.

Finally, an important professional issue – the individual teacher may be the first to recognize a child's difficulty in this learning area. In my view, they should take a step back before doing anything, as types of school and modes of engagement will probably dictate who should be told first. If, however, others know already they should have passed the information – in confidence of course – to you the teacher. Just because some music teachers are in schools for but two hours a week, there is no excuse for that information not to be given.

So, huge admiration for those who have fought through the odder aspects of musical organization as well as the challenges confronting musicians with this problem – or is it a gift?

Note: As indicated in the preface (p. xvi), the editors considered that at the end of some chapters it might be helpful if the book contained 'boxes' which encapsulated in the space of a few words some important insight. Except in the case of Chapter 6 they are not the work of the author whose chapter they follow.

> *If they don't learn the way you teach, can you teach the way they learn?*

Chapter 3
Dyslexia and musical development

VIOLET BRAND

Dyslexics have specific learning difficulties with written symbols in reading, writing and spelling. Unless these difficulties are recognized and the dyslexic children given the specific help they need the problems will not be overcome. Fortunately dyslexia is now officially recognized by the British government. Specific diagnosis and teaching are available in many state schools, as well as in the private sector.

Among the written symbols that cause problems are those of mathematics and music. This may be the case however gifted the child or adult is mathematically or musically. It is good news that increasing numbers of parents and teachers in Britain are becoming aware of the difficulties.

In 1971 Dr Macdonald Critchley, a British pioneer in the field of dyslexia, spoke at a conference in Sydney, Australia. In his lecture he said:

> The dyslexic child may also show difficulty with musical notation. The ambitious parent may try to get the youngster to learn to play the piano, and although he is keen and his co-ordination is adequate, he may find extreme difficulty in reading musical notation. (Critchley, 1971)

Subsequent events have proved him right.

How and when do these problems with music emerge? Often the child has enjoyed music, has been able to sing in tune before he could talk, and has a good musical ear and good musical sensitivity. So what happens?

When he is old enough (six to seven years) enthusiastic parents send him for piano lessons. For the first year there may be no problems. He plays the pieces beautifully, confirming the parents' claim that 'they have a musical child'. Then misery sets in.

First, he will not practise. Second, he does not want to go to piano lessons. Finally, he positively refuses to go to them. Everyone is puzzled, including the piano teacher. The adults think either that he is lazy or that his initial enthusiasm has worn off. Perhaps he was not as musical as they thought? They all remain puzzled, including the child himself.

The secret lies in those written symbols. For the first year he did not need to use them. The piano teacher played the new piece; the pupil observed where her hands were, heard the sounds (his ears told him about tune and rhythm) and he played the piece correctly.

Seemingly, too, his eyes were on the written music propped in front of him. This, however, was the problem: his eyes told him nothing! Just as the written symbols of words in books were preventing him from reading, so the written symbols of music finally halted his progress. In the first year his musical ear and sensitivity had carried him through, but after that the pieces became longer and frustration began to build up, until finally his music lessons, like his school lessons, became periods of failure.

Let us look at the specific problems. First, each of those 'wretched' notes on lines or spaces mean two different things – pitch (sounds – high or low) and time (length – long or short). Pitch symbols are named after the first seven letters of the alphabet. This presents a problem for dyslexics because they have difficulty remembering the order of the letters of the alphabet, and in the case of music there is a mixed order. In the treble clef the lines are named: E, G, B, D, F. If a child is learning the piano and using his left hand for the bass clef there are even greater problems as the lines are named differently: G, B, D, F, A. The letters represent the sounds of notes on the keyboard, but these symbols also represent time: the different lengths of sounds, long or short, are represented in music by different black or white symbols. It is difficult for the dyslexic to remember (a) what each symbol is called, and (b) what its length is. Why, after all, should a minim be called a minim? There is nothing about that small white circle with a tail that gives a clue to the name. Then, when that circle is black, it is called a crotchet. The dyslexic might remember that you clap one beat for a crotchet (♩) and two beats for a minim (♩), but it is the names of these written symbols that are the problem. Indeed, one of the central problems for the dyslexic is that of remembering the correct names or labels.

There is a further problem when words in a foreign language are used. Why should *andante* mean slow (at a walking pace) and *allegro* fast? When the dyslexic hears the music he will not forget which is fast and which is slow – it is those strange words that cause the problems.

However, foreign words are not the only ones that cause difficulties. If the piano teacher talks about the child's 'left hand' or 'right hand' he may be uncertain which is which! That is a hazard that not only applies to music, but also to games and learning to drive a car. It is important that the piano teacher (like the driving instructor) should *indicate* the hand, not just name it.

Any or all of these problems may affect the reading of music in the early stages and may prevent the musical youngster from continuing with an instrument, particularly if the difficulties that he has encountered have arisen from his attempts to play the piano.

A possible solution is to introduce the child to another instrument – one that requires only one line of music to be read. With the right teacher the child can then gain confidence and regain his or her enthusiasm. One possibility is that the child might take up a brass instrument, or perhaps the saxophone, or even the violin. If it is a low pitch instrument that appeals, such as the bassoon, then time will need to be spent helping him with the bass clef. However, if his chosen low pitch instrument is a saxophone or a brass band instrument then all is well – whatever the pitch. Pitch: the parts for these instruments are all written in the treble clef.

What about percussion? This is a question that parents of dyslexics often ask. There are hazards of which both the parents and the child should be aware. One is the organization that is required. If one observes percussion players at rehearsals or at concerts one will notice that they are often moving from instrument to instrument and from one sheet of music to another. Playing with a jazz band or a pop group without sheet music does not present the problems of playing with a classical group, wind band, or brass band: a dyslexic percussion player can have a marvellous time if he has a 'buddy' in the team who helps him to be in the correct place, at the correct time, playing the correct instrument.

An ongoing problem for dyslexics is that of sight-reading, especially at the speed required by the music or the conductor. In literacy a slow reading rate can affect dyslexics throughout their lives. This is now officially recognized, and they are given extra time in examinations. Extra time is also given nowadays in music examinations to any dyslexic candidates who have submitted a certificate. But for many dyslexics, despite the ingenuity that some of them show in working out compensatory strategies, the difficulties of sight-reading still persist.

Fortunately, as far as writing music is concerned, the technological advancement of music computer programmes has opened many doors, and gifted composers are able to get their creative thoughts accurately on to paper without worrying about how to get the music from their heads into written symbols.

Part of the enjoyment of music making is playing in a group. However, this can also present problems for the dyslexic: keeping one eye on the conductor and one eye on the music, particularly if this is a new piece, can be very difficult and can cause musical hazards. If the dyslexic can have new music before the rehearsal (perhaps a week, or a month) and practise at home before coming to play with the group, confidence and competence can be restored.

Singing in a choir, when this involves the simultaneous reading of both words and music, can cause further problems, particularly if the words are in a foreign language. Again, a possible solution is that the dyslexic singer should have the music well in advance of the first rehearsal.

Fortunately parents and teachers are becoming increasingly aware of all the potential difficulties. This means that it is now possible for musical dyslexics to be given the right kind of help, and where this happens there is every chance that they will overcome their problems and enjoy making music.

Chapter 4
The story of a dyslexic singer

ANNEMARIE SAND

There are two things that I always say when talking to people about dyslexia – that it takes courage to reveal oneself, and Einstein said that knowledge is experience and everything else is information. Both remain true for me.

I grew up in Denmark in a supportive family and with a twin sister. I was generally happy and fun to be with, until the time came (at age six) to go to school. Then boom! Everything seemed hard and I did not understand why I had to memorize everything in order to progress. It did not help that during this period of frustration my twin was fine and jumping ahead, whereas the skills that I mastered and stored, such as having fun, being joyful, being a great inventor and good company, were not important any more. My sister and I were therefore undergoing a major role change in our relationship as well as everything else. Things became confusing and it was very difficult to hang on to my own person.

At the age of about 10 I was tested (Denmark was in the van of the diagnostic tests in the early 1970s) and came out of school for three sessions each week to receive special tuition for two years. That itself created a number of challenges such as having to remember my route to the tutor, which buses to take in which direction, etc. On reflection I regard all that concentrated attention as an invasive process. The situation (not the remedial teaching itself) did a have a dark-tunnel effect, with a feeling that there was a world that I could not enter. 'I can't do what I should be doing: is there something wrong with me?'

After two years of this I had caught up on the spelling and language front but was behind in other subjects. I came to an interim conclusion that, generally, dyslexics are bright but have a problem organizing their learning. I also looked in the mirror and promised myself that I would catch up, and then the world would have to accept me on my own conditions. Towards the end of formal schooling I needed a break and decided to go to a sports school and have singing lessons as well. It appeared that entry to the Danish Music Academy would prove difficult as there was a tough requirement on the theory side, and it happened at that time that my twin sister was intending to come to England. After much debate about the wisdom of joining her in this adventure, but with my parents' backing, I did just that in a snowy 1979 and worked hard to gain entry to the Royal Academy of Music (performers' course).

Although many tutors were kind, there was no real knowledge of dyslexia or of how to spot its traits, and there were some periods when I felt 'down' and worthless. I did not tell anyone that I had these problems and just went about getting the information that I needed for my work.

I was happy with a new beginning in a new country. I found piano very hard work, but began to get high marks in singing. Fortunately high standards on the academic side were not required, and I was lucky to be offered many leading parts in oratorios, lieder competitions, and opera performances over the five years during which I was at the Royal Academy. (You really 'learn how to learn' only from doing it, not by talking about it). The choir was rather a problem – how to sight-sing with all that noise going on around you. I found a good solution: I always asked to sit next to the best sight-reader, and I could then sing to my heart's content.

All this experience was invaluable when I moved into the profession. Sometimes I had to ask for things that others did not need, like getting a conductor to promise to beat a particular passage more deliberately, or a repetiteur to spend more time with me than perhaps would be expected, so that I could really bank into memory a certain tricky page. Some of these learning strategies included asking colleagues to point out characteristics of a long sweep of music, for instance stormy accompaniment and drastic change of mood and orchestration. All these were an aid to memorizing, even though I do this mainly by picturing the music on the page.

I know that other professional colleagues think that there are many among them who have dyslexic traits in some combination or other. There is a sense that non-dyslexics are 'on the other side' simply because they do not experience our difficulties, but I dream of everybody being more open about these things.

In the family context I have found that simple musical strategies to do with memory and recall help the learning process with very young children, whether they are dyslexic or not. I have in mind such strategies as asking them to repeat the sounds that I myself have made, reminding them of previously sung fragments or intervals, and asking them to repeat them. It is associative, and I think it has a connection with my professional work.

I sometimes put songs or opera scenes into a grand 'aural-visual plan'. On a sheet of paper I might write in visual reminders of the musical milestones (changes of key or mood), or such musical characteristics as 'storm', 'darkness to light', or 'love scene'. I cannot, when performing, have recourse to the music text or to this 'plan', but it provides me with another source of reassurance; it is, of course, a multisensory device! Cues, general continuity, movements and my place in the whole scene are more easily remembered.

Sometimes people ask about approaches to foreign languages. It seems to me that dyslexics generally develop a great aural facility, so foreign languages themselves do not present a problem. It is the speed of reading that remains the hard part. Of course, as time has passed, I have worked out strategies (one aspect at a time, approaching the music from various angles, learning some things partly from tapes, and so forth) to help me along, and in whatever teaching that I do I try to maintain that multisensory approach.

The main thing is that I know how to learn my music and how to end up with a professional result. How I get there is not important.

What I say to people who are weighed down by dyslexia is this: being dyslexic has made me a very resourceful person. I really understand other people's points of view. In problem situations I can quickly see what is needed – the wisdom gained from having had to learn things from so many sides makes you very flexible. More importantly, I am not afraid of hard work to achieve my goal, which in the end is what matters.

I use my own individual symbols and pictures to remember articulation, expression and ornamentation.

Chapter 5
Some problems of a dyslexic flute player

CAROLINE OLDFIELD

We have all heard of dyslexia but has anyone stopped to think how this affects the musician? I can only tell you how it affects me. But bear in mind that no two dyslexia sufferers have identical problems, although it is likely that all will encounter at least some of mine.

Sheet music could be a lot of birds sitting on telegraph wires (instead of notes on a stave) for all the sense it makes to me. I have been taught F, A, C, E for the spaces and Every Good Boy Deserves Fun for the lines – which is fine for reading just the one note. But put more than one note or a phrase of notes together and the brain gets muddled and co-ordination becomes difficult.

It gets even further confused if the notes become dotted notes or are tied. This involves counting. What was an even rhythm is now a jerky one.

So here I am fumbling to find the right note and trying to count at the same time when suddenly an accidental appears – C flat or F flat or E sharp or B sharp. Now I'm really thrown off course. Why don't they write it as B, E, F or C? Quick, refer to the fingering chart on the front or back of the tutorial book and find out how to get that certain note. What do I find? The fingering is written as if one is playing a recorder, clarinet or oboe – vertically.

My problem now is to turn it horizontally in my mind – a task I find extremely difficult to do. If the flute is played horizontally why isn't the fingering chart also printed horizontally? My progress is even further hampered because the flute is unlike the piano (which I also attempted to play but only achieved Grade VI before admitting defeat). When playing the flute, to achieve the higher notes one works towards the mouth and vice versa for the lower notes. This is totally opposite from the piano and is just another problem to overcome.

Having sorted out the notes, their value, accidentals, fingering and expression, there now appears a further obstacle and that is leger lines – they all look alike to me. Thank heavens I don't play the piccolo!

At last I've managed to get to the end of the piece of music, an achievement in itself – now let's play it again just to make sure . . . I can't . . . because for all the good playing the piece through once has done I'm seeing it as if I'd never played it before – it might as well be a different piece of music altogether – so here I go again!

Only with constant repetition does something eventually sink in – but the danger with repetition is the music can become heavy and uninteresting, and this is something to be avoided at all costs. Therefore I would suggest 'little and often' and 'stop while everything is right'. To carry on only allows errors to creep in again, and once that happens you're back to square one.

My final obstacle in flute playing is that I forget which register I am playing in (although I can hear it in my head). This is because I have no 'fixed' point of reference. I'm not sure how to overcome this problem yet, but I'm working on it.

Maybe some of these hints that I've found helpful will also help other dyslexic flautists:

- first, avoid stressful situations – they only aggravate the problem;
- secondly, try to avoid pieces with too many accidentals (other than the sharps or flats in the key signature);
- thirdly, if it is possible, get the music enlarged. It helps to have the lines and spaces spaced apart more and avoids 'Is it a G or an A?' and so on.
- it helps also to have the G line marked in brown and Cs in yellow, and if you are playing the piano, the F line marked in red (as they did in years gone by before modern music printing took over).

We also need the patience, encouragement and understanding from our tutors, as we are not stupid – just people with a particular problem that is an invisible handicap. If only they knew how much effort has gone into learning a piece and overcoming the problems! Even half a page is an achievement, and to complete the piece totally is sheer delight and a joy to the dyslexic flautist.

Chapter 6
A personal view of dyslexia and professional music making

MICHAEL LEA

Learning about dyslexia over the last 12 years has been a liberating experience for me. It has enabled me to tap into a world of practical research. I have learned to produce handwriting that other people can read; I have learned to spell, and by reading slowly I have learned to read every word if need be, although I still enjoy my ability to skip through texts, hopping through the words. I have learned to memorize with confidence; I am learning the advantages of being able to slow down. With the use of a word processor I can write something and change my mind without having to throw away the paper and start again. This wastage had in the past been a source of great frustration for me and was very disheartening. By contrast, as a professional musician my difficulty with literacy skills was irrelevant; all I needed to do, other than play my instrument, was to sign my name and do my accounts.

It has always been a pleasure for me to sit down behind my bass and play. When I play my bass I am hearing sound and feeling vibrations: I feel the sound not just in my fingertips but throughout my body as I move bones and muscles to make the music. In addition there are many structures involved, from the structure of the music to the method through which I learned to play. All this multisensory and structured activity is focused on, and defined by, the music itself, which might be in any style.

Nobody knew about dyslexia at all when I was at school in the 1950s and 1960s. We muddled through as best we could, and perhaps were given more latitude than would have been allowed today. I attended Salisbury Cathedral School as a chorister and went on to Rugby School. Both schools now have advanced dyslexia units.

For me school life was fortunately much more than learning in class. Both my schools provided a rich learning environment outside of the classroom, as well as beautiful surroundings to grow up in. My twin interests were playing rugby football and playing music. At that time music was something that I did, whereas playing rugby was something that I worked hard at.

I learned to read before going to Salisbury, using Beacon Readers. I can remember learning to recognize the sounds and names of letters and learning how to put them together to make, at first, simple three-letter words, and then multisyllable words. My father was a minister and it was natural on some occasions to read passages from the authorized version of the Bible out loud with my parents, particularly from the psalms. I gained confidence working my way through the long biblical names such as Nebuchadnezzar. They were usually phonetic.

My first writing was legible and slow between two lines. The problems started to arise when I was required to write quickly. Over time I invented my own script, which was very fast. If I was not sure of a spelling I made every letter look the same. I can still read this script, although others can read it only with difficulty.

Learning by rote was always difficult for me. I knew nothing of sounding out loud what I needed to memorize. Indeed, in a room full of choristers, all doing supervised prep, this was impossible to do. Consequently reciting tables was a difficulty for me. Fortunately I had a good head for numbers and could calculate them as we went along. I had certain favourite numbers that served as bench marks, such as 'six eights are forty eight'. Learning vocabulary silently in Latin and French was impossible. Spelling remains a difficulty for me, though less so now than it was previously.

Another difficulty I had throughout my school life was that, although I became a voracious reader, devouring authors and not just books, I could never remember the answers to the questions likely to be asked in class, 'Who was . . .?' 'When did . . . happen?' These books had interested me in all kinds of ways, but recalling particular information on demand was beyond me then. I now know that I have a poor short-term memory.

When I was a chorister in Salisbury cathedral our life was always busy. We sang evensong six days a week, with three services on Sunday, 44 weeks a year. We sang a large repertoire from medieval plainsong to the latest offering from Benjamin Britten or Herbert Howells. It was cathedral policy to repeat very little in a year. We learned to sight-read. At first all this music went by in a mist, but after a while I began to find that I was catching on, and I became a good sight-reader. Perhaps singing in a group with the notes and bars going by at a set speed meant that those who had to read every note had to learn to keep up, whereas those, like myself, who skimmed through had to slow down in order to sing every note.

Choristers at Salisbury were expected to learn two instruments. I had piano lessons with different teachers. Every time I changed teachers I started from the beginning again. I was never very good, but I enjoyed playing the piano, particularly when, as a teenager, I accompanied my sister who played the flute. I learned to keep the time going and to sketch in what I could.

It was my good fortune at Salisbury to take up the 'cello when I was 11. Bridget Dearnley taught me in the traditional way, starting simply at first and adding in new techniques slowly one at a time. In the five terms during which she taught me I reached and passed Grade Five. This was effective teaching at a receptive age.

At Rugby I had many opportunities to play in orchestras, chamber groups and school music competitions. I was a member of a band that played at parties in the school holidays. Music was fun. The music staff, who were talented and enthusiastic, were the only teachers to give me good reports throughout my time there. One of my worst academic reports commented witheringly, 'I understand he is musical'.

I survived academically at Rugby by being in the top maths set, which guaranteed me one good mark. I was simply unable to produce consistent written work. The crossings out, the rewrites, and the illegible handwriting meant that it took too long to produce acceptable work. It was discouraging both for myself and for my teachers.

On leaving school, while I felt that music was what interested me most, I had no idea about what making a living from music entailed. However, I was accepted at the Guildhall School of Music. To start with I was overawed by the standard of playing, and I spent a term or two looking at other people's fingers out of the corner of my eye to see what they had that I hadn't. Was it the shape of their fingers that enabled them to play so impossibly well? Ken Heath took over as my teacher and taught me what I needed to know to make a living.

Ken Heath was very strong on the importance of building up neurological pathways. He said, 'You are learning to send messages to your brain in the most efficient way possible. You are learning to make these pathways secure and repeatable. Every mistake has a reason.' He counted a hesitation as a mistake. I was receiving thought-out, methodical teaching, and catching up fast. After a year at Guildhall I knew that professional music making was for me. I felt at home.

Towards the end of my second year at Guildhall, I realized that the sound in my head was that of the double bass rather than the cello. The size of the instrument was more natural for me, too. The changeover worked well, thanks to Jim Merritt, my bass teacher, and to the fact that the principles were the same. I had also learned how to practise effectively by then.

Memorizing pieces was still a problem for me on the bass, although on the guitar, my second instrument at Guildhall, I found memorizing easy and sight-reading impossible. Eventually I devised a process for learning to play from memory. First I learn to play the piece from the music. Then I re-learn the piece again completely from the beginning without any music. Finally I re-learn the piece a third time concentrating entirely on the interpretation, perhaps using a tape recorder to play alongside. This whole process can take a few days if it is a short orchestral solo, or a month on each stage if the movement is a bass concerto. I do this work on pieces that I can play through before I start studying them thoroughly in this way. Having put all this work in, I have a great respect for anyone who stands up and plays solos from memory in public.

I left music college as soon as I was offered a job, but I didn't stop studying. I studied extensively with many teachers, including Eugene Cruft, Adrian Beers, Tom Martin and Jean Marc Rollez. I was seeking out the knowledge that I needed and am grateful for their help. I also learned by sitting in bass sections and finding out what works by osmosis and by trial and error. Of particular use were the cello and bass classes that I attended, taken by Ken Heath and Robin McGee. In these classes a group of players learned how to make the bass line sound good. It was often the easy passages that required the most thought.

Learning about dyslexia was a revelation for me. I was in my late 30s when I was taught to write legibly for all to read. At last I had found an approach that worked. Using the techniques developed by Anna Gillingham, I learned cursive script, saying the actions out loud as I carried them out. I realized that it was possible to learn to spell by naming the letters out loud at the same time as I wrote them. I learned how dyslexia affects people in different ways, often with confusing and opposite results.

Once it was known that I knew something about dyslexia, many colleagues came to me telling of their problems – problems that seemed to me to point to dyslexia. I began to speculate that dyslexia in its widest sense is often present among professional musicians and their families.

The following are some of the points that occurred to me:

- It is said that dyslexic people are good at tasks requiring spatial awareness. Playing music clearly requires a high degree of spatial awareness.
- Looking around the orchestras, I found that these bright people, doing a highly complex multi-stranded task – that of playing music – often had academic qualifications much lower than one would have expected.
- The effective musical training that I had received seemed to me to correspond to the methods used in teaching literacy to dyslexics. The step-by-step approach pioneered by Gillingham and Stillman (1969) seemed to me to be mirrored in the traditional double bass teaching method books of Simandl (1964) and Bille (1922).
- Surely the act of playing an instrument, combining movement and sound directly connecting the tactile senses to the auditory senses, is 'multisensory'. 'Multisensory' teaching, as pioneered by Anna Gillingham, is a key technique for teaching dyslexics.

For myself, as I learned more about dyslexia I was able to make sense of much of my earlier academic failures and recognize my strengths. It was reassuring to find that there were others whose minds worked in the same way. My problems had answers.

Feel and sound are part of the same thing to musicians. They are what musicians add to the notes on the page when they are performing.

Feel is something that will grow of itself if you are aware –
Feel of the music; what gives it its style and sound –
Feel of the instrument; its weight, nature and materials –
Feel of warm hands, of breathing out –
Feel of the rough hair on the string, the stickiness of resin –
Feel of the slow bow-power.

Chapter 7
Silver lining

NIGEL CLARKE

To my son, Joshua, aged two and a half

Dear Joshua,

The dawn of a new century is a good time to reflect on the past and the future and learn the associated lessons. This letter tells you a little about my own past as a means of helping you (when you can eventually read it) to face the challenges of the twenty-first century.

It is my dearest hope that acquiring the skills to read this letter will not be so hard won for you as it was for me. As a young adult, I could barely read and assumed that I was stupid. I was aged 32 when I first found out that I was dyslexic. This was a decade after I had first met your mother, Stella. Stella had always felt there was something different about me, but did not know how to pinpoint it. One day she read a memo at work that listed the symptoms of dyslexia and exhorted recruiting managers not to write off applicants with these symptoms. Now she felt sure I was dyslexic and suggested that I visited the British Dyslexia Association to do some tests. I agreed and the rest is history.

We have no idea if you are dyslexic as yet. We are both prepared for this possibility due to the fact that dyslexia often runs in families, and having both become familiar with the characteristics of dyslexics we would view it positively. We would make sure that those in charge of your education understand. In my day less was known about dyslexia, and my difficulties in education were attributed to lack of ability or application. I understand that I was a disruptive child in primary school, and my parents recall one particular school report that said 'exasperating behaviour'! I failed my 11-plus exam (this was a state test which all children sat at the age of 11 to establish whether they were capable of going to grammar school) and went to the local secondary modern school. Secondary modern schools were there to train the less bright children to work in manual labour of some sort. I only ever managed to make one very crude aluminium ashtray during my five years of metal work classes! Ironically no one smoked in my family anyway!

The one subject I really enjoyed was music: I played the recorder in primary school and learned the cornet at secondary school. I knew that I wanted to take up music professionally from quite an early age. There was a history of brass players from my school going into the forces as musicians. Following in their footsteps I joined the Royal Marine Band service at Deal aged just 16. Within 18 months they had dismissed me for being 'unmusical'. The main reason was that I had a poor sense of rhythm, especially when reading music. I remember that learning to do military drill was hard. If I was not out of step, I would be turning in the wrong direction. It is difficult to know how bad I was – I was given three music exams, the idea being that if you failed all three you were asked to leave. After the first two failures, I decided that the machinery was in place to fail me, so, ignoring the standard criteria, I wrote my own exam piece. I failed. The Warrant Officer said that he had nonetheless enjoyed my music and that I should take it to an ex-colleague and friend of his, Peter Wastall. I did so, and for many years Peter encouraged my youthful attempts at composition without asking for any financial reward.

The practical realities of life loomed at this stage as I had left school without any qualifications to ensure employment. My only skills were the ability to play the trumpet and to work extremely hard. I entered the Staff Band of the Royal Army Medical Corps on the understanding that I was not of the right standard but that, if I worked hard, I would be supported. After a year or so of enjoying myself as a musician in the army I went to the Royal Military School of Music, Kneller Hall, and won the harmony prize. I was actively encouraged to write music by their harmony professor.

An early memory I have is of my parents stopping the car outside the Royal Academy of Music in London to have a look at this great institution. I dreamed of going there one day to study. The encouragement that Kneller Hall had given me fuelled this dream. The fact that I did not have any formal qualifications would occasionally bring me back to reality!

In 1981 my band was cut in the annual defence review and I faced the prospect of being made redundant. On a whim I auditioned for the Academy as a composer and, to my surprise, was accepted. I took the place without a grant. By sheer luck the Band of the Irish Guards, based in Chelsea, rang my Director of Music to say that they needed a trumpet/cornet-playing pianist of about my age. I was interviewed and was offered and accepted the position on the understanding that I would study at the Academy and be allowed one day off a week for study. This arrangement meant that my army wages would fund my studentship.

Going to the Academy was a major milestone. I studied with my hero, composer Paul Patterson, and it would be fair to say that for the first year or so I did not shine or respond to my lessons. I remember failing my first-year aural test and being summoned to the Director of Studies, who at that time was Christopher Regan. I thought this was the end of the road for me. Instead, Mr Regan was strangely supportive, saying that the Academy thought that I heard things differently from most people and that I should not worry but try to develop the skills needed to pass next time. I know now that my problem was my poor short-term memory.

One day the penny dropped! I felt at home at the Academy and began winning prizes including one adjudicated by Sir Michael Tippett. I was given scholarship and fellowship money to help me study. My greatest moment was when I was given the Queen's Commendation for Excellence for the best all-round student. This was the turning point for me. After this, there were still many more challenges, but I had proved that I could achieve the top award in one of the leading musical institutions in the world. A far cry from my dismal days at school and with the Royal Marines!

All the above may seem a rather sorry tale, but it is told in order to put my current position into perspective and to encourage you, who may also have the same challenges to face. From these difficult beginnings, I have now become a head of department in a leading music college, have five sets of letters after my name, as a composer have nine recorded CDs to my name, and am in the process of embarking on a promising film-composition career. I became the first associate composer to the Young Concert Artists Trust and I am currently the first composer in residence to the Black Dyke Mills Band. All this with the reading ability of a 16-year-old, the spelling ability of a 14-and-a-half-year-old, and the numerical ability of an 11-year-old!

It is true that I still feel uncomfortable admitting to having dyslexia because it seems like I am making excuses! Indeed, one might be tempted to use it as an excuse when it is simply the case that more effort is required. It is important to keep striving whatever the difficulties and to believe in oneself. Hard work and perseverance have played a big part in my achievements to date.

Clearly there is also an element of luck in everything; indeed our country's prisons are teeming with fellow dyslexics. I am one of the lucky ones. Being a dyslexic musician brings added challenge, as the whole music community is geared up to embrace genius and the most talented players and musicians. This means that you exist in an environment that does not encourage you to admit any type of weakness as this could potentially restrict opportunities that come your way.

My music reflects some of the problems that I have encountered en route. It is highly rhythmic which means my weakness has become my strength. Reflecting my approach to life, the music never gives up and always strives forward.

One of the major challenges I have faced working in education is adjudicating examinations and competitions. Here you have to be able to make notes and reports on the spot and any errors of spelling or grammar will be very obvious. I have found a number of strategies to overcome this including:

- Writing in advance phrases that I am likely to need so that these can be copied on to the examination or adjudication report.
- Taking someone with me who can write for me
- Writing the reports at home afterwards so that my wife can check them!

Dyslexia could be viewed as a life sentence – a sentence that condemns you to working harder than those around you, a sentence that means you always have to be on guard against those who might take advantage. On the other hand, it is sometimes said that dyslexic people have characteristics that can give them the edge in certain professions over non-dyslexics, for instance that they can think three dimentionally. I have indeed found that I can see potential ideas from all angles, and this helps me to visualise what needs to be developed further – a useful trait for a composer! I also put down to dyslexia my ability to organise and see clearly how a task or problem should be tackled. I am frequently amazed how people find the less than perfect route to solve a difficulty, and I believe that dyslexia gives me a 'helicopter' vision enabling me to cut to the heart of an issue.

Joshua, if you are dyslexic, we will see it as our role to help you discover what you are good at, and not to judge you by rigid and inapproptiate standards. We will expect you to put effort into developing yourself – we cannot do this for you. Above all, we will be positive and encourage you to use your talents in whatever walk of life you are best suited – perhaps even music!

As ever

Dad

Chapter 8
Books are my friends

JANET COKER

As a small child my idea of heaven was a new book. The feel of it, the smell of the glue from the spine, the wonderful pictures inside. It was a magic thing. I was the first person to see inside that book. The pictures were so clean and fresh and the colours like jewels. I could not read the words. My mother had to do that and if she was too busy then my imagination and the pictures were enough to make me very happy. I still feel like that with each new book I buy. I can read most of the words now, and my tastes are so wide as to encompass anything between soft or hardback covers – new stories, the history of the world, the imagination of millions of human beings, the thoughts and ideas of different cultures for us to explore, all between the pages of a book.

I also love the look and feel of a new piece of music or a new music score. To hold them gives me the same thrill – the excitement of discovering stories in sound, the thrill of expressing all the emotions mankind is capable of feeling. The sheer beauty of music feeds the soul and lifts the heart.

All over the world people are reading books and making music. You can't make war while making music.

But when it comes to opening that new piece of music or that brand new score the shock is profound! No pictures, no clues – terror, frustration, anger that I can't reach the music. I know it's there as I have heard it and seen it performed. Other people can interpret these dots, lines and squiggles. Anger, anger! Why can't I?

While writing all this, I have realized just how much books are my friends and music scores my enemies. They were things that I had to fight, to battle with and conquer before I was allowed to sing. No wonder it has been so hard.

But I must change that thought – I would like music scores to become my friends, just as books are.

Chapter 9
Continuing to sing: a postgraduate view

PAULA BISHOP

As a dyslexic person I have shared in the many frustrations and challenges that a conventional education brings. Music has always played a central role in my life: from a young age 'singing' and 'I' became intertwined. I continued along this path, deciding to go to university before postgraduate study in singing; and I am now combining a practical singing course with a master's degree at the Royal Academy of Music (RAM). I was not assessed as being dyslexic until after I graduated.

The RAM has taken many initiatives to help with its understanding of matters such as dyslexia. Alongside my own practical and academic work in music I have found much joy in teaching both these aspects of music to pupils of various ages, whether dyslexic or not. The combination of all three of these areas – practical work, academic work and teaching – has culminated in a wish to study music and dyslexia at the doctoral level. I would like briefly to explore some of the shifting challenges that I have found in following this career.

As I struggled through primary school, music was a refuge from written language. My teachers enabled me to discover and nurture my aural abilities for learning and self-expression. Although I could read music as a result of learning the piano – a continuing battle to this day as I found it hard – I preferred not to do so. It was this freedom to improvise and to use my aural abilities that gave me confidence and enjoyment in music. Now, as a teacher, it makes me sad to see the emphasis placed nowadays on examinations in every subject; the result is that children with their individual needs and learning strategies are forced to become 'standardized', and if they do not comply they are labelled failures. The confidence that music gave me from an early age had two main results. First, when I had to start working hard at my music, as I had to if I was to be successful, I already knew the joys of performance – I had experienced the feeling of success and emotional satisfaction, with the result that it was something worth working for. Secondly, because my confidence had been built up, the result was that I was able to perform and express myself. I realized that words, when combined with music, were not quite so scary. This increase in confidence was first brought to my attention when I won a creative writing competition at the age of 6. The head teacher had no idea how to read my writing and so asked me to read it aloud to the school. This could have been the most embarrassing moment of my short life, but instead I remembered the ideas instilled in me by my father: putting over the meaning of a song and not being embarrassed. In fact I made up another story as I could not read my own!

I continued with my singing at the secondary stage and was able to take my General Certificate of Secondary Education (GCSE) in music a year early. This gave me another confidence boost. I sang in many choirs and music groups, and had singing lessons. In addition to having my confidence built up as a small child through music, I also had the rare opportunity to be exposed to other ways of learning than those that were given to me at school. I won prizes for singing and found myself in the company of composers, singers, conductors and instrumentalists who came to music, and possibly more importantly to literature, from another angle. I shall always remember the composer Robert Saxton coming to sit by me at a rehearsal. I was trying to choose a poem to recite for my Guildhall audition the next day. I was leafing through a book of Yeats, and Robert Saxton started to discuss the possible choices. Treating me as an equal, he spoke with such enthusiasm that I felt myself drawn up into a world that I had previously found impenetrable. I was not being taught in the conventional way, but I was learning more and wanting to learn more than ever before. I could see links between music and the rest of the world – history, literature, art, politics. These were the connections that I needed to make in order to maintain any sort of enthusiasm for the written word.

As I seemed to be embarking upon the early stages of a career in singing, I became increasingly aware of the emphasis that musicians put upon the reading of music – sight-singing and the ability to learn music from a text. There was always a feeling that if you used recorded material to help the learning process you were in some way an inferior musician. It has taken me many years to re-evaluate this matter and to start using recorded material as a valuable resource. Also, as a teacher, I try to instil in my young pupils that text is not music – it is a means of storing and communicating music. It is only when we *perform* the music that it becomes alive; notation is there to aid us, not as a barrier to expression. If we place too much emphasis upon text this deprives us of the opportunity to explore to the limits the boundaries of our musicality. One of my most precious memories is as a 16-year-old singing my first real operatic role – Flora in Benjamin Britten's *The Turn of the Screw*. I had learned the role, and after a few days of rehearsal it was my big moment to sing Flora's solo, a haunting lullaby. The conductor asked me to improvise the melody and possibly some other words rather than sing it straight. I was scared – but let myself go and sang something. The whole room was silent and I improvised for three minutes or so. At the end the conductor just said, 'I think we should write that in. It was beautiful.' That was one of the few times in my musical career that I really expressed what I wanted to say – a rare thing for anyone but even rarer for a dyslexic person whose modes of expression are often more limited. It also proved to me that music could be a channel for words as well as notes.

This channel is unfortunately limited to words in my own language. Music is one of the few arts that uses many foreign languages – instrumental music as well as the obvious vocal lyrics. This continues to be a concern for me and for many other singers. I have learned to love words in my own language but it took much longer to gain that appreciation for other languages. As with all aspects of my life, I have been fortunate to have found inspiration and help from a mentor. While I was an undergraduate, my French teacher, who was trying to teach me French for the fourth time, would read me French poetry explaining the landscape of emotions, not the grammar. I learned to love the sound of the language and for a moment stopped seeing the collage of letters and sounds.

My final thought stems from combining all these thoughts on expression, improvisation and so on into something more tangible and practical. Those of us who have managed to break down the barriers to music and have chosen a career in it are still faced with the everyday trials of being dyslexic. If you are capable and organized, as you must be, even those who know you are dyslexic do not really understand what that means: to them you do not 'seem' dyslexic. Situations arise in everyday life, however, which present you with problems. For example, you are handed a 30-page document in a meeting and are asked to make intelligent comments on it during that meeting. My point is that we have a long way to go before an invisible difficulty such as dyslexia has the same recognition as, say, being blind. Having a problem with reading is still in some ways associated with lack of intelligence. This is something that we are trying to correct, for if people want our insights, which are many and varied, it is important that we help them understand how they can get the best from us.

As I struggled through primary school music was a refuge from written language.

Chapter 10
My experiences as a dyslexic musician

O<small>LLY</small> S<small>MITH</small>

I began to play music before I knew I was dyslexic. When I was aged 8 my parents suggested that I learn an instrument and so the recorder seemed a good one to start with. Twelve years later, the recorder – as well as a music degree – is a major part of my life.

Until very recently I never really considered that being dyslexic would greatly affect my ability to learn music. However, I realize that I have been very lucky, having been equipped with a generally very good education and with sympathetic teachers and lecturers. At primary school I was academically well behind most other children, but I was very fortunate to go to a good prep school when I was 8 years old. Within a year the school had realized that I had a form of dyslexia. As a result I had two years' extensive individual tuition from the Dyslexia Unit in Winchester. I basically re-learned how to read, write, and spell using the phonetic, syllabic, and visual systems. Without this individual and specialist help I do not believe that I would have been able to have attended university or coped as a musician.

I initially learned to play and read music almost exclusively through my individual recorder lessons. At prep school I fortunately did not learn the recorder in a group in the classroom as it could have confused me and put me off playing the instrument. In group music lessons I could not and still cannot grasp or under-stand the system of 'doh, ray, me'. However, even at an extremely early age I had a passion for listening to music. Even at prep school I could understand and recog-nize the different kinds of music better than most other children. Some of my earliest memories were of music, and I can still remember lying in bed at home, listening to my father's record player from downstairs, and falling asleep to the gentle hum of a Beethoven symphony.

I developed very slowly as a musician because for the first few years I found reading musical notation difficult. However, I never felt frustrated and did not notice that other children were progressing more quickly than I was. There are probably many reasons why I did not give up the recorder even though it was a struggle. It was mainly because I was, and still am, a determined person and will never give up. In fact my non-dyslexic twin brother had recorder lessons with me for about six months and he actually gave up having lessons. It was probably too difficult and too much hard work for him, but it certainly motivated me to carry on playing!

I also did not notice that I was initially learning the recorder very slowly. Although other children at my school were learning other instruments I did not meet another serious recorder player until I was about 16 years old, and only then did I realize that I was about two years behind other recorder players of my own age. However I eventually caught them up with the help of good recorder teachers.

Looking back, I believe that my dyslexia may have contributed to my slow progress on the recorder. Remembering fingerings and notes was not too much of a problem as I remember fingerings quickly by relating them to patterns, but I found it difficult to understand and read rhythms, and co-ordination between the tongue and fingers has always been tricky. With persistence I have managed to acquire most of the necessary techniques, and I know of non-dyslexics who also find such techniques difficult.

By the time I was taking my General Certificate of Secondary Education (GCSE) music exams I could cope very well with the academic and theoretical side of music. I really enjoyed GCSE Music because it was fairly practical, with a wide range of subjects and a broad genre of music. A-level Music was a lot harder, but I grasped the history of music very quickly and can remember facts and dates quite easily. I also did well with my coursework essay, even without any extra help. However, I did extremely badly in the written exam and struggled with tonal harmony – and even now I cannot spot consecutive fifths and octaves!

Luckily, at university in Bangor, I have no exams for the present and have mostly good lecturers who have re-taught me how to do tonal harmony with a completely different system. In brief, I prefer to work with figured bass rather than the traditional 'Vb' type of chord indication, which involves a mixture of letters and numbers. I strongly recommend all musicians, including dyslexics, to learn some figured bass, especially if you find playing piano music very difficult. I myself struggle to read piano music at speed but find it easier to grasp a Baroque keyboard part with figured bass. Originally keyboard continuo parts had only a bass line with figures, and once you get to know the figures you can construct your own chords within this framework.

What I like about Renaissance and Baroque music is the fact that there is a lot of improvisation. As a recorder player I do not have to play exactly what is written on the page. Actually most composers of the time encouraged performers to individualize the music by cutting notes short or making them longer. The music is also bare and without ornamentation, and sometimes a piece of music becomes so elaborate that the performer is like a second composer.

I also find the individual interpretation of early music fascinating and great fun. The advantage about it is that I do not need to write down my own ornamentation to the exact demisemiquaver (32nd note) and can actually remember an awful lot without having to write much down. I think this is where dyslexic musicians are at an advantage because many non-dyslexics I know have to write out absolutely everything. I am hopeless at mathematically writing out even a simple trill or turn, but I can play one without thinking about it.

I think a lot comes with practice, persistence and patience, and I do not think saying you are dyslexic is an excuse when you cannot do something first time. I find it really hard work to play the recorder well. I have a lot against me as the fingering is illogical; it takes years and years to produce a good sound, and it is extremely difficult to stay in tune! However, most non-dyslexics find the recorder just as difficult to play well and the only major difference, I think, is that a non-dyslexic will grasp new techniques quicker than a dyslexic person will. But in my own time, and with persistence, I can usually catch them up!

A lot of dyslexic people complain that sight-reading is extremely difficult. I know I am only mildly dyslexic but I have found a very good way of counteracting this. At every recorder lesson, my teacher and I sight-read duets. I do not have time to prepare and instead have to read at speed. You do not have time to worry about individual notes and instead you can concentrate on not getting lost! It is usually a bonus if you can work out what a D-double-flat is, but, as you are sight-reading at such a speed, usually the fingers take control of the notes. The brain can then concentrate on keeping time and watching that I am co-ordinated with the other recorder part (i.e. I have to read almost two parts at once). When it comes to practical exams, a piece of sight-reading seems relatively easy as I have to read only one line of music; I usually have time to prepare, and I feel under less pressure because I know – having to read only a single line – that I shall not get lost!

This kind of sight-reading helps me to improve my counting as well as confidence. Instead of counting triplets and crotchets mathematically, I feel them. Many musicians, whether dyslexic or not, are not too good at counting. My recorder teacher tells me to use a metronome, but I feel that the only way I can learn really complicated modern music is an extremely slow way. Sometimes I have to copy it out and learn it by ear and repetition from my teacher, bar by bar.

I think it is sometimes a poor excuse to give up on something and blame it on genetics, dyslexia or a disability. I know a good folk musician with Parkinson's disease and a professional harpsichord player who translates his music into Braille because he is blind. If people can play music well with a physical disability, then I think it should be possible for those with dyslexia. I use my own individual symbols and pictures to remember articulation, expression and ornamentation. I should be lost without a pencil because, if I work hard on a piece of music, then it is usually thick with pencil markings to prompt me to play music in my own interpretative style as well as getting the notes and rhythms right. It may look incomprehensible to other people but this does not matter as long as I understand it!

I think that dyslexic people struggle with general organization. I have acquired what I think are some reasonably efficient strategies for surviving at university. First, I must look after myself. This may seem simple and obvious enough, but I know students, dyslexic and non-dyslexic, who do not sleep or eat much, or keep fit and healthy. Sometimes a five minute nap is really refreshing if I am tired and stressed. I am also lucky that I can cook and enjoy doing it.

Once you have coped with this, it is easier to become organized in other ways. I have a terrible short-term memory, so I write little notes (memos) for myself so as to ensure that I do not miss a lecture, rehearsal, work deadline, or train. These notes are then left in strategic places around the room. My room has to remain tidy, with everything off the floor, so that I know exactly where everything is. That way I do not forget or lose things, and it stops me from becoming frustrated and wasting time trying to find things. It may sound strange, but I have a corner for practical music books, manuscripts and recorders and a corner for my clothes. Important and urgent things, such as work to be submitted or letters to be posted, are left on the floor so that I trip up on them and do not forget they are there!

If I am in a rush and late for something (as I usually am!) then I can also pick up a piece of music or work instantly if I know where it is. However, what does frustrate me is that some publishers of music insist on having exactly the same colour and font design for their music manuscripts. I have at least ten pieces published by one publisher and they all have identical orange front covers. It is very annoying: I discover that I have picked up the wrong piece of music for a recorder lesson in Manchester – say, the Telemann sonata in place of the Telemann concerto – and I cannot pop back to Bangor to retrieve it! I wish more publishers would use different colours and fonts for the front covers.

In any case I think dyslexic people have to be extra disciplined. Thus I find that I cannot spend my afternoons in the pub and expect to write an essay in time for a given deadline. Although friends of mine can work all night and complete the essay minutes before it is due to be handed in (and usually get annoyingly good marks for a last-minute essay!) I have to take twice as long to achieve a good result.

Many people in choirs that I have been involved in cannot actually read music but they cope with singing and enjoy it. I feel nervous when singing on my own, but in a group I can sight-sing fairly well. Singing in a foreign language is not usually too much of a problem, except if that language is German! This is because I learned to read syllabically and syllable division in German is very difficult. In the case of Welsh words I have learned their pronunciation through singing Welsh songs even though I still cannot understand the language. Sometimes I am at an advantage compared with non-dyslexic people as I can sing in Old English and grasp the meaning straight away!

I can also relax and learn plenty from folk musicians in pubs. Many folk players are better musicians than many classical musicians are, even though some of them are musically illiterate. Instead many folk musician rely on the oral tradition – they learn tunes by listening to each other.

However, if you want to play classical music then I think you do need to learn traditional Western notation. Perhaps the only answer is practice and persistence, unless you can invent your own form of notation like Braille, figured bass, or guitar or lute tablature. However, learning the treble clef should not be too difficult and a mnemonic such as 'Every Good Boy Deserves Football' helps you remember the lines on the treble clef. For the order of sharps I still have to remember 'Father Christmas Goes Down And Eats Breakfast' (the order of flats is the same thing backwards).

Practice and persistence do eventually pay off. I still struggle to understand and remember foreign words for performance directions, and I probably take longer than most musicians to grasp even simple techniques. However, I do not complain or blame it on dyslexia when I do not achieve something easily. Equally, I am not ashamed or embarrassed about being dyslexic nor do I wish to hide the fact. I may find music hard work, but even the most talented musician would (or should) admit that they are still learning to improve as a musician. Dyslexic or not, very few musicians will agree that music is easy to play well and comprehend. But without the challenges I certainly would not be a musician or a recorder player.

Chapter 11
A struggle to play

Jacob Wiltshire

I love music. I love playing, composing and listening to music. My favourite instrument is the guitar. Until now I have only been writing music by ear but now at school we are learning to actually properly write music. OK, I am all right in maths and history; my spelling and reading have improved tremendously in English, but in music I find myself lagging behind. I can't keep up! It's so annoying to see everyone else playing fluently and poor old confused me sitting there with my keyboard wondering what to do next or what key to play next. Every time I look at a manuscript paper it's just like reading some alien language written in 'ds' and 'ps'. A fuse in my mind blows – something in there wants to leap out and start playing a Mozart symphony or even *Frère Jacques* – at least something. But no! Instead I find myself staring into a piece of paper, trying to work out what this means.

It's like trying to find a picture in one of those magic eye things. You know it's there but for some reason you can't find it. It's a struggle to keep going, especially when everyone around you is laughing and talking to each other because they cracked it ages ago, and you're still struggling with pain in the mind to read this stupid piece of paper with black and white drawings on it. It is very helpful having a mum who is very sympathetic and she has a board with plastic notes on to help me, but it is still like a snail trying to complete the London marathon – because all I want to do is write music and perform.

Note. This was written when Jacob was aged 11. Eds.

Chapter 12
My experiences with the problem of reading music

SIW WOOD

I was born in 1934. In my young days dyslexia had not been recognized. My mother was a doctor and extremely impatient with me. I can remember her saying when I was about 6 or 7, 'I cannot understand why this child cannot read – I cannot remember a time when I could not read.' I was told that I was stupid both by my parents and by my teachers – until I believed I was. By my teens I had an outsized inferiority complex that lasted well into my 40s.

At school, some time between the ages of 8 and 12, I can vaguely remember that a rudimentary explanation of how to read music was given to me, but it did not 'go in'.

At the age of 12 I was sent to a Quaker boarding school and I expressed a desire to learn an instrument. It was decided that I should have violin lessons (because my parents had a violin that had belonged to my uncle). As I had a good ear I made progress and got through the whole of Book One of the exercises and simple tunes simply by copying the notes the teacher played on the piano. She had not enquired whether I could read music; she had just assumed that I could, and I was far too inhibited to tell her I could not.

One lesson into Book Two I played my first wrong note. 'What note is that?' she said. I made a wild guess – 'B'. 'No, of course it's not, you stupid girl.' There ended my violin lessons.

I have always loved singing (Welsh ancestry). Starting at school, I have sung in choirs virtually all my life. However, I always have immense difficulty learning words by heart.

The music 'goes in' and stays. I have a good ear, as I said earlier, which enables me to pick up the notes and memorize them very quickly. I also have a good sense of rhythm, so, unless it is very complicated, the rhythm 'goes in' too, although I am not good at counting as such.

God compensated me for being dyslexic by making me a top soprano; as a result I am helped by the fact that the soprano line is the top stave. I would find it

51

very difficult to look up at the conductor and then down again to find my place if I were an alto. I use a highlighter to make sure I can pick out quickly where I am on the page. However it is very difficult for me to find my place when the music requires me to turn back for a repeat, and I have to mark the place with huge arrows.

If I am given a relatively simple piece of music (one without complicated runs) I can sight-read it accurately even if I am unaccompanied. I know the value of notes by their appearance but might not be able to name them correctly. I know where middle C is on the stave but still can't name what the other notes are without laboriously counting up from middle C. I understand sharps and flats.

I started having singing lessons, with the hope of doing some solo work, at the age of 50. One teacher said, 'Oh! I'll teach you to read music – no problem!' But she gave up willingly when I expressed the view that too much of the lesson was being taken up with this and not with vocal technique. She even tried to teach me mnemonics to remember the names of the notes on the treble and bass staves – but I could not remember the mnemonic either!

Now my biggest difficulty is learning the words of songs by heart. I struggle if the words are English – if they are Welsh it is virtually impossible! I put them on tape, and listen and listen and stare at the page, and repeatedly mutter them again and again, day after day. Sometimes it gets to the point when I can sing along with the choir OK, though I would be unable to sing the words solo. For the National Eisteddfod no copies of the words are allowed, and I suffer all sorts of panic feelings – hoping that the conductor does not stop mouthing the words, as she usually does.

As a solo singer I cannot feel safe without the words, written large, on a music stand so that I can glance at them. There are a few songs, usually simple ballads, that I learned at school and can still remember. I think this is partly because a ballad paints a mental picture that runs in my mind like a film.

I can remember things that form mental pictures. People ask me if I have read a particular book, and when I look doubtful they name the author, which is of no help! If, however, I ask, 'What is it about?' and they start telling me, then once I have heard the start of the story I have no difficulty in saying whether or not I have read it before.

If all a child can see is difficulties in symbolic notation the other aspects of music will be lost. Notation is there to aid us not as a barrier to expression.

Chapter 13
My music and my dyscalculia

HELEN POOLE

My music at school – problems and compensatory strategies

Is it any wonder that children with both diagnosed and undiagnosed dyslexia or dyscalculia have a fear of school and of academic achievement?

The belief that 'seek and you shall find' is of little comfort to the dyslexic or dyscalculic student who is left to struggle unaided in the whirlpool of symbolic language. My mother and brother, to whom I am eternally grateful for their persistence and patience, spent hours of frustrated battle with me in an effort to get me to 'see' how easy it was to learn my times tables and other 'elementary' mathematical topics such as long division, long multiplication and converting units of measure into other units. I was often seen as a 'wilful' child who closed her mind to what was being said, and so my teachers were reluctant to tackle these problems or find ways of helping me to learn. I began to work out my own compensatory strategies.

All was not rosy on the music side, certainly as far as systematic and sympathetic teaching was concerned. This left me at a great disadvantage as music was both my ambition and passion, and I was unfortunately forced to lead myself down a rather solitary path in the quest for gaining musical knowledge both in and out of the school environment.

As I became older and my passion for music became more intense, I turned my back on all those who had jeered at me for not possessing the right kind of 'knowledge' of music or, in their eyes, potential for musicianship. I tried instead to become my own music teacher, formulating my own rules and going at my own pace.

Having spent years being criminally led to believe that music was one very complex unit that only people in the school bands were able to do, I hope that young musicians like myself who were shunned at school for not grasping the ideas of music theory and applying them to 'musical knowledge', will be given full reward and credit for their perseverance.

For me, no one could ever deny me the uplifting feeling of an instrument that rested in my hand or lay snugly on my lap. Children are praised for their performance in a test or in a sports race and are pushed to becoming the best academics they can be. Why does the child who spends hours of blowing, bowing or strumming never hear the songs of praise for his or her efforts or dedication – even if he still is apparently making the same 'dreadful' noise as yesterday?

Since I began to learn to play musical instruments at secondary school I have been guided by the principle of first listening and playing by ear before reading musical notation.

It was when I progressed to the graded systems of assessment and examination and began to play in youth orchestras that the problems with my ability to learn musical theory really began to show up. I was seen to have 'great problems' in attempting certain areas of music, namely those that involved skills exclusively needed in examination-type situations. A clear example of my inability to succeed in the graded musical system occurred when my trombone teacher suggested that I do my grades four and five. I soon found that I had no chance of passing the examinations because of the poverty of my aural test skills. These tricky tasks included:

- repeating back a line of melody played on a keyboard (I ended up forgetting the start of the piece before it was finished).
- sight-reading sheet music. (In this task I used all the designated time to work out what notes I ought to be playing and where on the instrument, and determining the key, and then I did not have any time left to work out the rhythm or time signature. I became very flustered because of my awareness of the short time available, and had 'sensory overloads' where I became completely mind-blocked and useless. I always failed these tasks miserably.)

I found that trying to master aural test skills at the last minute before an exam was impossible. However, in the music lessons that I was given in the class it was assumed that if you could play well there would be little difficulty in these areas, and so there was little time given over to practising them.

I found that 'little and often' never worked for me – it needed to be 'lots and often'! I was never made aware of my achievements in learning to play my musical instruments. The teachers and other students seemed just to focus on all the problems I had. Among the most important were:

- becoming seriously discouraged when required to read musical notation;
- becoming frustrated (the dyslexic person may have to make twice the effort of a non-dyslexic person, and may practise long hours while achieving only half the result);

- writing out music accurately;
- learning and remembering the correct sequencing of scales and arpeggios;
- sight-reading or sight-singing music;
- transposing music or reading different clefs.

I have arrived at my nineteenth year with the ability to play several instruments, mainly by self-teaching, even though I remain musically 'illiterate'. I attribute this learning partly to experimentation on my own and partly to close observation of the fingerings and techniques used by others and listening to the sounds that they produce.

Since leaving school I have shied away from very rigid orchestra systems, as there was no real room for individuality of playing or experimentation. Rather than try to memorize written musical notation I try to remember visual patterns that my fingers can then play.

So one could say that I have little choice but to 'feel' the music instead of being bound by a sheet of notation. I can read music – after years of relying on sayings ('Every Good Boy Deserves Food'), though when I try to work out which finger to use I am very slow. This is because I seem to be counting the spaces between the lines on the stave and each written note, and then I have to count the same number of spaces between my fingers on the keys of the piano or the slider on the trombone. On hand-held instruments such as the flute, saxophone or guitar I cannot apply this method, and because of my slow progress in learning to read the notation I continue to play by ear.

I have found that I do not automatically know what note-letter to associate with the key or button that I have to press on the instrument, but I can hear the tone that will come out of the instrument if I press a certain key or move it in a certain way. The problem of learning 'paired associations' between musical symbols and their names is exactly the same as that which arises when numeric symbols have to be paired with their names.

As I continue to compose today, more often than not I simply record musical ideas on to audiotape and use my musical 'ear' to 'find' the right notes if I have forgotten any of them.

Only now do I realize just how much I used to just leave things that I didn't understand first time off so as to keep up with the class. What I should have done is ask for clarification or explanation.

Having the time to practise on my own meant – and still means – that I can walk away if I get flustered. My piano teacher would never accept that I needed time to think in silence about what I was about to play. If I played a wrong note I needed to pause before attempting to correct it – I needed the time to work out where in fact my fingers ought to have gone.

The future

I have always been a very advanced speaker and reader and a 'bright' A/B grade academic student at school, and it has only recently been discovered that the root cause of my almost unbelievable problems throughout school in my maths and music (and also in history dates, geography bearings, and so forth) was the handicap I now know as dyscalculia. The various problems I encountered both at home and at school I can now see as part and parcel of my undiagnosed dyscalculia.

Dienes (1960), the mathematics teacher responsible for devising Dienes blocks, has said: 'Mathematics is a structure of relationships, the formal symbolism being merely a way of communicating parts of the structure from one person to another.' The learning of mathematics is basically, in my view, the learning of such structures. Music, too, has a structure, and the problem for the dyscalculic musician is that of learning the notation in which these structures are conveyed.

Hubicki and Miles (1991) call attention to the difference between the *sounds* of music and *musical notation*. They suggest that a knowledge of musical notation, though not absolutely *essential* for the appreciation of music, can greatly enhance one's understanding and enjoyment of it. They suggest that in the teaching of both music and mathematics there should be 'doing' first (playing music, adding and subtracting solid blocks to and from each other) and that explanation of the notation (crotchets, 'plus' signs, and so forth) should come afterwards. This seems correct to me. As I would put the matter, the aim of the music teacher should be to share with pupils the magic of the music itself and take as much time as is necessary for explaining to them the basics of musical notation and theory. If all a child can see is difficulties in symbolic notation, these other aspects of music will be lost.

Chapter 14
John and his cornet

Sylvia Gilpin

His school told us he was reading, yet John did not know his alphabet after more than a year at school. Fortunately a knowledgeable friend advised us to have him tested by an educational psychologist who found that, although he was very bright, he was dyslexic and a non-reader. He already believed he was stupid at age 6, but with specialist dyslexic help he was soon reading beyond his years. He attended a school that greatly valued musical accomplishment. However, we had observed that academically able pupils were chosen over others to play an instrument. We decided not to wait to see if he would or would not be offered an instrument, but to enrol him right away at a Saturday music course that his sister, not dyslexic, already attended.

We had already observed that the brass teaching seemed especially lively at the Saturday course. The head of the orchestra, a brass player, let John try out several brass instruments and decided that a cornet would suit him best because he was on the small side. We mentioned to the teacher that John was dyslexic in case that might affect the choice of instrument. He replied: 'Some of my best pupils are dyslexic.' We never looked back.

John enjoyed playing tremendously. His teacher followed a very structured approach with lots of repetition and praise. From almost day one he insisted that John should join a beginning orchestra. John was extremely proud of his accomplishments and when he joined the Scouts he took a music badge and played a solo in front of a large audience. By the time he reached junior school he was more advanced musically than most other pupils his own age and was 'invited' (rather than auditioned) to join the school orchestra and band.

By the time he left primary school last summer he had taken Grade Five and had played several solos to great applause at school events. He had also joined a local education authority orchestra and band that meets several times a year and has already played at the Royal Albert Hall and at the Camden Jazz Café.

Taking his grade examinations has been a reasonably relaxed process for him to date because his teacher has helped him to prepare well. He has not had to learn too much theory yet. Sight-reading, however, has not been easy for him. He began learning to play the drums about a year ago, and this has undoubtedly helped his sense of rhythm. At home we have gently encouraged him to practise. His father, especially, has played a crucial part in encouraging his progress and has accompanied him on the piano at each examination.

The move to secondary school a year ago has been a big change for John. The school is some way away and he leaves home very early in the morning and returns just before supper. He has to do homework and this makes music practice hard to fit in. Although the new school has several bands and a music department, John has not taken to this. None of his new school friends plays an instrument.

Although John continues to go to the Saturday music school, he is becoming resentful of this after a long week of school, especially when his new friends invite him to go out with them on the Saturday. We have compromised by reducing the time from half a day to two-and-a-half hours and allowing him to miss some Saturdays. He says he feels his trumpet teacher pressurizes him to continue and that he really does not like playing the cornet. He has hardly practised at all between lessons and does not wish to take any more music examinations. During our recent summer break he said, 'I have only just remembered that I play the cornet'

We are in a quandary about his future studies. Whether because of pressures at school (perhaps arising from his dyslexia) or for some other reason, he is at present in a rather unsettled state. It may be that he is on a plateau after his very good progress until age 11 and that he will come back to music at a later date.

Chapter 15
The piano tuner

GILL BACKHOUSE

At nearly 70 years of age, Philip remembers all too well one way in which dyslexia affected his school days. Up on the board would go the hundreds, tens and units sums. He would call out the right answer and then write it down wrongly – '235' for 'two hundred and fifty three'. Whack! 'Idiot! Careless boy!' Although he was a slow reader and often missed letters out when writing, problems with numbers seem to have been the greatest frustration.

Philip, however, could sing like an angel and longed to play the piano and have lessons from Miss W, the Sunday School teacher. He often accompanied his mother to houses that she cleaned and knew of a small, neglected piano at one where the owners had been kind to him. Without his mother knowing, he persuaded them to give him the piano and (aged nine) managed, with the help of the local policeman, to get it home on a barrow. When his mother came home and found it in the front room she was not pleased and he got a beating. The piano stayed, however, but as Philip started to pick out tunes he knew it didn't sound right. Soon he was inside the frame fiddling about and realized that the strings needed tightening if it was to sound like the one at school. Grandpa was persuaded to make a gadget, to the boy's design, which much to his satisfaction 'worked a treat'. Philip tried his best to earn the eightpence a week needed for piano lessons by walking a neighbour's dog, but never managed to reach his goal.

During the war, Philip was sent to live in Wales with his maternal grandmother. Here his musicality was recognized and encouraged by his teacher, who both sang and played the piano himself. A new pupil with such a voice was a joy for the musical Mr. Jones. Philip sang in eisteddfods all over Wales and realizes now that his ability to sing anything once he had heard it, and also to harmonize effortlessly, probably masked his inability to read music accurately or know a fourth from a fifth on the stave. Philip's forthright comments about pianos that did and didn't 'sound right' did not pass unnoticed during this time.

Philip was 13 when he returned to London and joined the local army cadets as a drummer. The bandmaster (a graduate of Kneller Hall), irritated by Philip's restlessness at the first practice, enquired why the boy kept turning round. 'Something sounds wrong, sir.' He was marched between the rows of instrumentalists till the trouble was identified – a 'mismatch' between bugle and trumpet (inherent in the nature of the two different instruments). 'If you can hear that, lad, you have a fine sense of relative pitch.' Philip was then invited to join a small 'orchestra' at the bandmaster's house where various instrumentalists met on Sunday evenings to play for pleasure. He found the tenor drum 'didn't sound right' and set to, tuning it until it was perfect all the way round.

Philip left school at fourteen and, after an unhappy interlude in his father's shop, found himself a job in a piano factory where he learned to build and tune pianos. This was not the same, however, as a proper apprenticeship and he had no opportunity to go to college.

He carried on playing in the cadet band, becoming drum major, and when only 16 was placed seventh in the drum majors' section at an all-England band competition. On the strength of this and a recommendation from his bandmaster, his two years of national service were spent in a regimental band.

Philip's faultless sense of rhythm and practical ability served him well when marching, but his persisting difficulties with sight-reading, despite several years of near continuous music making, made orchestra playing problematical. Unlike the other musicians, he needed to look at the score beforehand if he was to get through orchestra practice without making too many mistakes. Once again the cocky young Philip drew the attention of his superiors. He was not afraid to say if he thought other instruments were out of tune – much to the annoyance of older hands. He would arrive well before afternoon rehearsals began, to study the scores and tune his 'timps' to perfection with a tuning fork . He was right about his fellow instrumentalists on more than one occasion and finally told to 'wipe that cheeky grin off your face' – and transferred to Kneller Hall! His posting there was a short one – after two months he was returned to his regimental band. His sight-reading problems too often led to mistakes that could not be tolerated – cymbal and drum reversed at the end of a phrase quite ruined the effect. He recalls being tested time and again during the weeks before he was finally ejected from this most famous academy, but that nobody tried to teach him to follow the score accurately or to question why he still could not do so, despite the fact that he had been playing and singing since he was 11.

Following demobilization Philip returned to the piano factory and continued to learn his trade. He subsequently established himself as a tuner with a large round of loyal customers, and as a successful businessman restoring and dealing in high-quality instruments.

Many years later, when his mother moved house, Philip found all his old school books and reports in the attic. His wife noticed that the many answers to his maths problems marked with large red crosses were in fact correct but written back to front. 'Didn't your teachers notice?' she asked. It was then that Philip, with the help of his wife, began to realize that he was probably dyslexic. He recalls the rage he felt (and still does) that his teachers could not see that there was something wrong – rather than a careless and wilful boy who 'could do better'.

Philip says that he could 'get the gist of crotchets and quavers' – just like written words, in which he perceives rhythm at every turn (Waterloo, Victoria, Elephant-and-Castle were tapped out on the table when explaining this point). He particularly recalls thinking, when he was stationed in Germany, what splendidly complex rhythms were evoked by local polysyllabic place names. (By coincidence, PM, the subject of 'A Pianist's Story' in Chapter 19 of this book, uses words to fix rhythms in her mind.) In Philip's opinion every child should learn about rhythm before learning to read, as this would help them to tackle longer words. (The results of years of academic research support his view!)

Philip's message to every parent of a musical child is this: expert, one-to-one help from a sympathetic teacher must be sought at the first sign of difficulty. A teacher must be found who is willing to try to understand the child's needs and adapt his method – not just carry on as usual.

Philip's passion for music of all types has never dimmed and is far from passive. When he hears music he cannot sit still. He sings and conducts, or taps out the rhythm (he remembers using knives on the kitchen table as a child). The emotion evoked in him by music is clearly intense. During our interview, tears sprang to his eyes as he recalled the high spots of his musical performances as a boy soprano, humming the melodies of much-loved pieces. Poverty may have prevented him from having those longed for piano lessons as a child, but at school and in the army there was considerable opportunity to master sight-reading and be part of a wider musical scene. The route to a career as a musician was, however, blocked by his problems with musical notation – a difficulty in automatically accessing the vast repertoire of music played at concerts every day. He is constantly reminded of his dyslexia by the many errors he makes when transcribing customers' phone numbers – an irritating tendency to reverse numbers which he sees as an exact parallel to the problems he had when he used to reverse the last two notes in a bar of music.

There seems a real possibility that, had someone noticed Philip's difficulties and succeeded in helping him learn to read music, he might have pursued a successful career as a professional musician and enjoyed a lifetime of making music with others. As it is, despite his many achievements, he is left with reminders of what might have been. In his own words: 'OK. I may not be able to play the piano, but I'm a bloody good tuner.'

Chapter 16
Teaching the piano to Deirdre

DIANA DITCHFIELD

This chapter is a record of my experiences in teaching the piano to one individual child. I offer it in the hope that some of it will strike 'chords' (if I may use the pun) with other music teachers.

I first started teaching the piano to Deirdre in 1993 when she was aged just 6. Several observations led me to suspect that she might be dyslexic. In particular:

- Her concentration span was very short – it was not easy to persuade her to sit still on the piano stool for more than about 30 seconds.
- Even at the end of playing one bar of crotchets she had more difficulty than most of her peers in remembering the first of the four notes that she had just played – she could neither name the note nor say where it was on the piano; it seemed as though she had somehow 'blanked out'.
- A videotaped lesson in 1994 showed that although she was able to identify and play middle C on the stave if this was what the stave indicated, when she was presented with the notation for middle C in a new piece she asked what was the note's name. This seems to be an example of the difficulty, experienced by most dyslexics, of associating symbols with their *names*.
- Progress was unusually slow for a child of her age and vitality. Her frequent singing suggested that she was no less musical than her peers, yet she needed more time than they did to learn a new piece and, having learned it, she needed more time to make her performance secure.
- More than most children whom I have taught, Deirdre would switch from one hand to the other to play a note. As far as she was concerned, it didn't matter which hand played middle C, regardless of the clef instruction in the printed music. Although it would have been my normal practice with most children to call attention to this, there was something about Deirdre's performance that led me to decide not to pursue the matter – perhaps because I felt that it would have added to her stress for only a small amount of gain.

- In contrast I was left in no doubt of her intelligence. In particular she could make imaginative connections, which she was able to explain clearly and in a lively manner. For example, when shown a picture of a church organ she immediately suggested that there was about to be a wedding! In addition, the pictures in her music book were always a source of much interest to her and she frequently decided that they needed embellishment.

Teachers, in my experience, can often arrive at a 'hunch' that a particular child is dyslexic and is different in subtle ways from children who, despite difficulties, do not present as typical dyslexics. This is what happened to me after a short period of working with Deirdre. Overall she seemed to me to be showing the curious *imbalance* of skills that one reads about in the dyslexia literature. Despite her relatively slow progress at the piano and her difficulty in remembering the name 'middle C' (see above) she clearly had artistic gifts and the ability to think imaginatively.

My own interest in dyslexia had come about in 1984 as Director of Music in a small public school in the United Kingdom. I also taught English to a small class of pre-GCSE girls, many of whom had been diagnosed as dyslexic. At the time it seemed to me that the girls who were in the chapel choir were making better progress in English than those who were not, and I wondered if this was because choral training helps to separate the syllables.

When I tentatively mentioned to Deirdre's mother my suspicions that she was dyslexic, a smile came over her face. She told me that there was a local centre for helping dyslexic children and that Deirdre had been going there for a couple of months. The programme for teaching her the piano was primarily driven by the required curriculum of the school. What this involved in Deirdre's case was to proceed as far as possible, step by step with frequent repetition, just as is the practice in the teaching of literacy. The acquisition of literacy – including literacy in the field of musical notation – needs to be a structured and cumulative process involving a large amount of repetition. It needs to be 'multisensory' in that all the senses need to be involved: the learner needs to look carefully, to listen carefully, and to pay attention to the movements of the mouth in saying words and to the movements of the hand in writing them. Just as an inexperienced person may find it helpful to try out the sound of a word with the aim of trying to find a match with a word that is already familiar, so a music student may try to 'proof-read' a succession of notes so as to check if they 'sound right'. As teachers of reading and spelling know, the kinaesthetic sense can be very important; similarly in the learning of a musical instrument there has to be training of the 'muscular memory'.

One of the ways in which I was able to offer support was by helping her to play notes steadily and rhythmically. For example, if she needed to play the notes C, E, and D in slow tempo I would not only *name* these notes for her but accompany her playing of them with a steady count – 'C two three four, E two three four, D two three four'. Deirdre found this very enjoyable, and of course it provided an instant check as to whether she was playing the correct note. I suspect, too, that it also helped to improve her sense of rhythm.

The motor control required for playing the piano causes problems for most learners and, of course, for dyslexics in particular. Constant practising is needed if results are to be produced which sound musical. There is a possible parallel here with physical education, where even seemingly clumsy children can learn to improve the ways in which they execute movements.

A common characteristic of dyslexics is that they are often afraid of making mistakes. This, of course, is not surprising, given that in the classroom they frequently *do* make mistakes – not only over spellings but over such things as arriving for appointments at the right time. What I noticed about Deirdre was that she seemed to become abnormally stressed when confronted with the unknown, for example on the first occasion when she had to play a new piece. In general, my suspicion is that insensitive handling on the part of some teachers, although it is entirely unintentional, may nevertheless contribute to the stresses with which dyslexics have to contend. In Deirdre's case I found it particularly necessary to be positive and encouraging and not to 'nag' her.

Her problems over concentration meant that it was necessary to find creative ways throughout the half-hour lesson of sustaining her interest and enjoyment. I sometimes had the impression that I was playing a see-saw with Deirdre: each of us accommodated the other more than would have been necessary for most children of her age and musical ability!

She enjoyed songs and could sing in tune, so I gave her the opportunity to add some of her own words to the pieces that she was playing. For example, when she played a piece that contained four bars of regular crotchets and happened to see a picture of some cartoon men going up and down a hill, she sang 'These men go right up – two, three, four: then they go right down – two three four'. And she was clearly enjoying herself!

Given that the learning of musical notation was difficult for Deirdre it seemed particularly important that she should perceive her lessons not simply as a 'grind' but as an opportunity to enjoy the things that she could do well and show her teacher how well she could do them. To give her an additional incentive, it was decided to enter her for the first of two house exams run by the school (Associated Board, pre-Grade I). At this time she was aged six and a half. Her first attempt resulted in disaster. She tripped up the stairs on the way to the examination room, which was not the best of starts, and when she reached the examination room things went from bad to worse: she bumped into the piano, slipped off the edge of the stool, and ended up so that she was not opposite middle C as she had expected. As a result she lost her bearings and started on the wrong note. She knew it sounded wrong and she panicked, but was unable to correct herself. Not surprisingly she failed. On her next attempt, however, she was not only successful but obtained honours. When I spoke to her afterwards she agreed that this was ample compensation for the traumas of her first attempt!

Now one cannot, of course, say with certainty what were the factors that led to her improved performance. However, an event that could have been significant for her was that during the period between the two examinations she was given an assessment and a 'statement of special needs'. As a result of 'statementing' the authorities are required by law to try to meet the needs specified in the statement. If this is done with sensitivity it can sometimes lead to a great improvement in the child's self-confidence. In Deirdre's case, for whatever reason, the success in her music examination was also accompanied by considerable progress in other areas. Thus she did extremely well in an elocution/drama competition; she passed tests of swimming and of Irish dancing, and the school reported that her ability to socialize was much improved. We cannot be sure what is in store for Deirdre in the future, but since she has a supportive home and most of her teachers are well informed about dyslexia there cannot but be grounds for optimism.

Conclusions

What, then, can be learned from my experiences with Deirdre? Certainly it is clear that dyslexia need not be an obstacle to a child's learning the piano – and that even the notation of music can be mastered if the teacher proceeds slowly and steadily. It is sometimes said that having to deal with information on two staves as opposed to a single stave presents difficulties for dyslexics; but it is clear that in Deirdre's case the difficulties were not insurmountable. The benefits to any child of learning to play a musical instrument need not be argued here. Quite apart from all these, however, there is, in the case of the dyslexic learner, the added factor of increased self-confidence. Despite their difficulties with memorizing musical notation, dyslexics can be sensitive musicians, as Deirdre was, and, above all, if they have sensitive teaching they can learn to *enjoy* music – both making it and listening to it. Seeing this enjoyment can be very rewarding to a teacher.

(On musical games, by Katie Overy.)
Musical games can provide a fun, non-threatening environment in which children can learn and practise as they play; an opportunity which is important for children who may be experiencing failure and frustration in many other areas of their schooling.

Chapter 17
The dyslexic chorister

SHEILA OGLETHORPE

The information in this chapter has been culled from 33 choir schools and from five other cathedrals, or centres of worship, which provide choral services for the community on a daily, or near daily, basis. At least 37 dyslexic choristers currently singing in cathedral choirs have been identified.*

During a normal week the average number of hours that a cathedral chorister works *in addition* to ordinary school hours appears to be about 21. In the case of the choir school chorister the week usually begins on Monday morning with a choir practice for an hour at about 8 a.m. On a weekday there will be another choir practice for an hour or so before evensong, which itself is likely to take about 45 minutes. Altogether the chorister will be performing his duties, either in choir practice or in church, for about three hours a day from Monday to Saturday. On Sundays the demands will be even heavier.

Besides offering sung worship almost every day of the year there will be ordinations, civic services, weddings, funerals, memorial services and concerts. There may be live broadcasts as well as recordings and there will inevitably be choir recitals. Everything needs rehearsal.

In addition, however, a chorister is often an instrumental musician in the making and will almost certainly be learning to play at least one instrument, often two and sometimes three. This means that he will have at least one lesson on his instrument each week and need to carry out the requisite practice. He is also likely to be in demand for a school orchestra and often for a chamber music group, both of which may rehearse once a week on a regular basis.

One may begin to wonder how the chorister fits any academic work or games at all into his daily timetable. He has to be extremely dedicated and so do his parents. Being a chauffeur to a chorister can be hugely demanding in terms of time!

---

* Because of the preponderance of boys among the choirs of these cathedrals the chorister is referred to for simplicity in what follows as 'he', although dyslexic girl choristers are certainly known today and probably will continue to be part of the cathedral scene in years to come.

Some headmasters have a policy of not even considering a dyslexic boy for a choristership. They feel that the demands made on choristers are too great for a child who has other problems as well. On the other hand there are headmasters who, provided that the child's difficulties are not too crippling, are very ready to take dyslexics. They feel that a poor performance in stringent academic tests at age 7 or 8 should not stop children with vocal ability from becoming choristers. His choral scholarship is likely to last for about 5 years – from the age of 8 to when his voice breaks, probably at 13, when he will move on to his senior school. These are five crucial years in a child's development, not only as a musician but in the classroom.

So all will depend on the headmaster. If he is willing to consider a child with learning difficulties (which can sometimes be hard to spot, especially if he is still very young and has not been at a first-rate infant school) he will need not only faith in his special needs department, but also faith in the potential commitment and motivation that he has noted at the child's interview. He will also have recognized that spark of intelligence that many a dyslexic child often projects in conversation, and his experience of the changes – sometimes quite dramatic – that can happen to a child when life as a chorister begins will reassure him that the risk is worth taking.

Having won through and started as a chorister, any child's life completely changes. For a dyslexic these changes are enormously important, particularly for his self-esteem.

First he is accepted. It is recognized by everyone, not just his own family, that he has a special talent that the majority of other people do not have. Immediately there is somewhere where he belongs and a group of his peers who know he has gone through the same rigorous tests that they went through at their auditions, and that he too has come out with flying colours.

Secondly, possibly for the first time in his life, he is treated as a professional right from the start of his choristership. The situation has its downside, as will be seen, but nevertheless respect from other people – be it ever so subtle – is, as everyone knows, one of the vital steps towards achieving a feeling of self-value. Parents have spoken of 'getting their child back', after having previously witnessed a steady decline in his opinion of himself to the point where he has consistently maintained that he is 'rubbish'. Other more belligerent children, when constantly belittled by class teachers, have adopted an 'I'll show them' attitude, and their frustration, which earlier may have resulted in disruptive behaviour, has almost miraculously disappeared when their musical talent has been recognized and respected. It is also likely to be very important to a child's parents that he is respected. Many parents get weary of making excuses for their son's poor showing at anything academic, and they worry about his future. When he becomes a chorister and his musical talent is openly recognized and acknowledged, it is as if a light were turned on in a dark room. This emotional relief at the turn of events helps the boy: he senses his parents' pride in him and it gives him status in the family, which, however hard his parents may have tried to persuade him otherwise, was probably missing before his choristership.

Thirdly, he is now among a group of boys who enjoy singing as much as he does. For him, as well as for most of them, music is meat and drink. He can empathize with them and he no longer feels lonely. His social skills can begin to blossom in a way they never did, and never could have, among his peers at his primary school. More often than not he also has to board, which can help him to develop socially and make him more self-reliant and mature.

These, then, are the three factors that reverse the downward progress of his self-esteem and help him to feel that he has something valuable to contribute. Few children of 7 or 8 will go so far as to analyse what they are feeling about themselves, but the adults in charge of them soon notice what is going on. The immediate effect of a choral scholarship can be very positive and encouraging.

The road to ultimate success in terms of a happy, well-balanced 13-year-old can, however, be extremely hard. There are those dyslexics who do not really reap the full benefits of their chorister years until they have left them behind. The pressure of work throughout the day is relentless and many a child is swept along in some kind of mild nightmare for his first year or two, being told where to go and what to do from minute to minute.

At the beginning, when he is a probationer, he will often be looked after very carefully and reminded of everything he should be doing, both by a member of staff and also by a more senior member of the choir. As time goes on he will be expected to remember for himself. He is not on his own, of course, because there will be an intake of several probationers, but the dyslexic chorister is likely to be the only one with a short-term memory problem for speech, which as a consequence gives rise to disorganization and lack of concentration.

There is no room in a choir for someone who is totally disorganized or who does not concentrate. These are difficulties that the dyslexic has to learn to overcome or circumvent in some way, at least while he is in the choir. Much can depend on his peers: they can be very kind and helpful but this is not always the case. The dyslexic is not free from the possibility of being bullied and having to suffer taunts, even when he has achieved the status of chorister. Choristers are thrown together for a large percentage of their time. They see more of one another than many families see of each other and sometimes at least one of them is unsympathetic. Making friends outside the choir can be difficult because the time the chorister spends with the choir is the time that his non-chorister friends will be spending with each other. It is a simple logistical problem.

For the most part it seems that choir members are very supportive of one another – they develop an understanding of the panic that some of them, particularly dyslexics, experience at times. They get to know and accept one another – they have to – and it is this unspoken acceptance, coupled with his own individual spark, that helps the dyslexic chorister to rise above the taunts that he almost inevitably will meet in the early days of his choristership.

One of his strengths is likely to be his ability to reproduce and memorize sounds accurately, particularly if they are not too complex and he is regularly exposed to the same ones. This is what sees him through the different settings of the services, the psalms and the anthems. Gradually he will begin to know almost everything from memory. His reading during the practices and services is all related to pitch and when the psalms, for instance, come round regularly once a month, as they mostly do in Christian churches where the choir is resident during term time, the repetition helps to familiarize him with the words. The special educational needs teacher in at least one choir school helps her dyslexic charge by running through the psalms for the day with him, familiarizing him with the words and their pronunciation.

What the dyslexic often finds most difficult is carrying things out at speed. This can be very alarming to the child who needs plenty of time. Nobody is going to stop for him to sort himself out or work out what the words are. It is not in the nature of music to stop; and even during the singing of the psalms there is a subtle speech rhythm to which he must conform. Moreover choirmasters set themselves a very tight schedule and do not have the time to make sure that every member of the choir knows exactly what he is doing.

Many choirmasters insist that every chorister follows the text with his finger. This is a practice that is very helpful to the dyslexic, even though at first the speed may come as a severe shock to him, and in spite of everything he may get lost. This practice is, in fact, a form of paired reading, which is advocated for dyslexics in the classroom, but it has the added advantage of helping them to associate words with pitch. In the psalms the pitch will change, more often than not, at the bar line, and the end of the line of the metric hymn is easily recognized by the tune. These indications in the text are of great assistance to a child who might otherwise be easily lost. It is even possible that they may help him to look out for punctuation when reading in the classroom. What is clear is that dramatic improvements in reading and tracking skills have been achieved in the first year of a dyslexic's choristership – so much so that choirmasters can sometimes forget that there was ever a problem. Of course, they do not see the bizarre spelling, the sometimes untidy handwriting and, in some cases, the difficulties with mathematics or French that are often all too obvious in the classroom.

Nor does it matter to the choirmaster or to the dyslexic chorister if he does not understand the meaning of the words that he is singing. A choirmaster will do his best to explain – albeit cursorily at times when he is under pressure – and the organist will colour the accompaniment to match the mood if he can, but a chorister does not have to be dyslexic to have little comprehension of what it is all about. Often when a dyslexic has only mild reading problems it is his comprehension of what he has read that is at fault. Many a parent has mentioned that their son concentrates so hard on getting each individual word right that when he comes to the end of the sentence he has no idea what it means. He has to read it through two or three times in order to comprehend it – the words and how they relate to each other getting easier each time. He may, however, sing straight through several psalms in a row without knowing what the words mean, but as long as he has sung the right words at the same time as everyone else in the choir it matters not to him nor to the choirmaster. He has done his job satisfactorily in that regard.

Some dyslexic choristers may need to wear tinted lenses or to use tinted acetate sheets, not only to help counteract the glare of white paper, but also to calm the eye muscles, thereby preventing both words and notes from apparently jumping around the page. Acetate sheets can be a great help but their disadvantage is that sometimes they tend to reflect the light, making the situation worse, and when a many-paged anthem is being sung they have to be moved too often for comfort. Tinted prism glasses are often the answer and can have a remarkably beneficial effect. It would probably help if a child with visual problems were also allowed to use copies with larger print, although this might be a bit of an administrative nightmare.

Some dyslexics find difficulties in adjusting from the blackboard to the book in front of them. In the cathedral read 'conductor' for 'blackboard'. For some dyslexics, constant adjustment from near to far can be especially tiring, and it may take a long time for them to get used to watching the conductor while keeping their eye on the text. It is often the case that as a result of constant reminders from the choirmaster the boy eventually does his best to learn all the standard repertoire from memory. He is left with the problem of less known and new works, but by the time he is fairly senior in the choir he may also have developed his own strategies for coping.

It is very rare indeed to hear of a dyslexic chorister who was not able to stay the course, though for some it has been an enormous struggle. One of the worst problems has been that of concentration, which has sometimes led to acute tiredness and even illness. The headmaster who suggests that it can be counterproductive to accept dyslexics into the choir has a point where the boy who suffers badly from poor concentration is concerned. Undoubtedly his concentration improves through his work in the choir and when he is singing. It has to – he is aware of that – and the motivation is there for him to improve. Outside the choir he may not improve to nearly the same extent. The immediacy of performance is within the choir – the next note, the next bar that everyone must sing together – but he has a perception of what concentration is about even if he cannot hold himself to it when he is on his own doing his homework.

One of the advantages of the training that a chorister receives is the ability to work to deadlines. Concentrated rehearsal for a performance of some sort – perhaps for a choir recital – starts only about a week, at most, before the event. The choirmaster may have 'nibbled' at the work or works for several weeks beforehand, but when work begins in earnest there is no room for lack of concentration. The dyslexic often fails to perceive the passing of time (which may come in useful during sermons!) but it would appear that something in the chorister's life has a beneficial effect on his ability to be ready for the occasion. It prepares him for the last-minute rush and helps him to produce reserves of concentration just when they are needed. Conversely, it does nothing to discourage the habit of leaving everything to the last minute – which also has its drawbacks!

Dyslexia manifests itself in many different ways and to varying degrees of severity, so it would be unwise to generalize about the overall success that a dyslexic achieves during his career as a chorister. It seems clear, however, that dyslexia is not an insurmountable bar towards becoming head chorister, which is a responsible position. Dyslexic head choristers are known, although they are relatively rare. Only one boy in each year can be head chorister anyway (barring voices breaking before the year is up), but many, if not all, are given the opportunity to sing solos in their final year or two, and it is in this area where the dyslexic is often a real star. Headmasters and choirmasters alike have commented on the beautiful voices and the impressive musicianship of some dyslexics and have said how pleased they are that they took the risk in admitting the boy in the first place.

There are many moving stories about dyslexic choristers told both by their parents and also by choirmasters and headmasters. They are stories of determination to win through in the face of very real difficulty, in demanding circumstances, and they speak of hard work and character in a way that is most humbling. They also speak of ultimate success in terms of stardom in the choir as well as music scholarships to secondary schools and often success in the professional world of music.

While researching this chapter I was sent two letters and a short story from which I should like to quote some extracts. These extracts perhaps go some way towards illustrating not only the feelings of rage, frustration and despair, of futility, vulnerability and confusion that many a dyslexic child faces, but also the ultimate release that becoming a chorister can bring about. The sender was James (not his real name):

Dear Mrs Ogelthorpe
I am a dilexic chirister at Z— Cathedral. I have been hir for Nealy a term and a harf. I like singing we do good music at broadcast and on memebance Sunday. We have just had a Xiat where we get to go hom for the weakend. In the Christmas holiday I went to test for tinted glasses. On Saturday of our Xiat I got my glasses and the first Evensong I did I washt aloud to use them. But Now I am.
    If you would like to hear from Me Please call me sometime in half term

I wrote to James and also got in touch with his parents. He had been admitted to the choir when he was already approaching the upper age limit for admissions, which in this case was rather older than at most cathedrals. His choirmaster had already been in touch with me and had affirmed that James had an exceptional voice but that he had difficulty with the pointing of the psalms. He was very well motivated and he knew that he must concentrate. His parents also wrote enclosing a story that James had written before becoming a chorister. The following are extracts:

AT the waters edge
Sam was backward, well that was what Mrs Tunse his form teacher ex army soldier bellowed at him. Now the chilldren were looking at him like a tiger in a zoo. Slowly he picked up his pen a red hot angry felling and a cold shivery icy sad felling rushed over him, leaving him wrapped in a blanket of fear terror sandnes. He wrote a few letters then dropped his pen, not able to carry on. His dinner was cold now and Sam felt sick

He through his dinner off the table shot off tearing the horrible blanket off him. He ran untill he got to the beach and he walked to the caves where he so often sat talking with the sea. The sea meant so much to him it would comfort him when he was sad, share his joy when he was happy, and most of all it was the only person who didn't critisize him. Tom picked up a stick and with great difficulty wrote in the sand:-
'I hafe the worLb' – which means 'I hate the world'.

He must have stayed their for hours . . . he did have a watch but he couldn't use it. So he stayed their untill he was sure school had finished. He walked back to school and sneaked in so the caretaker wouldn't see him, picked up his bag and ran out to get the bus home.

Sam walked in through the dor of his house 'Where have you been' asked his mum 'weve had evrybody looking for you' 'promise me you will Never do it again'

'I think he's heard enough' said dad camly.

When he went to school the next day he got a right earfull from Mrs Tunse 'Youre 11 she screamed you can't even look after yourself. you cant even right your letters the right way round'.

'Now chilldren sighed Mrs Tunse a new boy called Jack is coming today. put your hand up if you'd like to be his freind'.'Howabout you Sam see if you can do anything right'

Jack was sat with Sam. Jack saw Sams work. 'Your dislexic ar'nt you Sam.

His mother wrote:

In addition to his obvious literacy problems James has always had poor organisational skills and during his first half term at Z— he struggled. For example, he could not read or follow his timetable; he went to a clarinet lesson without his clarinet and lost two coats! Since then he has made huge strides forward: he now knows the sequence of the days of the week, and, furthermore, knows what day it is and what happens on that day. He has also learnt to tell the time. I think that the structured and disciplined life of a chorister is very beneficial to him.

Because he is dyslexic he has to rely heavily on his ear; his sense of pitch, of blending with other voices and musical expression is well developed. He gets a real 'buzz' from singing with the full choir. The first time I visited him, nine days after the beginning of the September term, I felt that he was complete. The jigsaw piece that had been missing all his life had been slotted into place.

Two weeks later the following letter arrived from James:

> Dear Mrs Ogethorpe
> Thankyou for your letter . . .
>
> It is frusttrating having reading difficulties but I don't want to give up paticully when we try out for solos and I can't read it.
>
> I like singing with the men best because I can learn from them by watching theme and listening. I like concerts better than sevices because the musics better . . . Music gives me a confidence boost because school is hard. Music Art games and story writing are my strong points. I like shakespere.
>
> The hardest things for me are German Geography and maths. My teachers for geography and maths don't no what it's like being dyslexic.
>
> I really really wanted to come to Z— because I wanted to do music and because it's the best school we come to.
>
> Being a chorister has given me great satisfaction and confidence. I do music every day and I can't imagine being with out it. Things I find difficult because I'm dyslexic are
>
> 1. the pointing in psalms muddles me up
> 2. I find it hard to look at the conductor and then find my place again in the music
> 3. Sight reading
>
> Things that Im good at because im dyslexic are
>
> 1. Imagining things
> 2. Listening
> 3. Knowing and feeling what the music is going like
>
> Not only have I had help with this letter from my freind and my mum but the outher boys In the choir also help me with reading and my music and augernising it.

I salute him.

Postscript:

It has just been announced, at the time of going to press, that James has been selected as a finalist in the BBC Young Chorister of the Year 2000 award.

Chapter 18
The dyslexic at music college

Margaret Hubicki

Dyslexic music students who wish to study at one of Britain's music conservatoires will almost certainly find that suitable provision is made for them. The understanding and support that is available is always towards helping to remove the barriers that can prevent students from achieving what they are capable of – not to do with lowering rigorous standards. Naturally some students may feel very sensitive about letting it be known that they are dyslexic. Their apprehension can include a feeling of 'doors being shut against them' – that they may be penalized in some way, particularly if earlier experiences have already brought disappointment.

Due to a growing awareness of dyslexia and its problems, such matters as these are being addressed and dealt with at music colleges. However, no help is possible unless those in a position to offer it are made aware of a student's needs. Information about these needs must clearly come from the student himself or herself in order to alert staff – no one can expect the authorities to be aware of their dyslexia by a kind of second sight! It is particularly sad when a student has suffered much and realizes too late that help would have been available from the start had it been sought.

The exact details of the provision for dyslexic students are constantly under review and naturally vary from college to college; the common aim is to meet the individual needs of each student. Information concerning the steps that have to be taken in order to obtain help is part of the material sent by the colleges with their application forms or after acceptance. In some cases the student may be eligible for funding to pay for specialist equipment or for formal assessment by an educational psychologist (see below), while in some cases the college will already possess equipment that could be helpful – at the very least word processors and technology for transcribing sounds into musical notation.

Applicants will usually find that the college staff are willing to try to answer questions about specific problems, and an important aspect of the colleges' policy is to try to remove fears on the part of dyslexic students that the authorities will be aware only of the 'negative' side to dyslexia. The students can counter this by the quality of their performance.

The nine major conservatories have contributed information to this chapter or concurred with its general outline. Much of what is set out above is probably true of most Higher Education institutions (compare Gilroy and Miles, 1995; Singleton, 1998). There appears to be a trend for students to ask for greater clarity from the institution about its policy on dyslexic-type difficulties. Exactly how the system for tangible assistance works may change over time. The avenue *at the moment* is for the student, if deemed eligible, to be awarded a Disabled Student's Allowance (DSA).* Negotiations for this take place between students and their home local education authority (LEA). A recent assessment from an educational psychologist or other suitably qualified person is usually asked for. Grants are made according to the pattern of dyslexic traits and can be quite generous – particularly as regards the provision of information technology hardware. Grants are not means tested, although it appears that they are not normally available to postgraduates. Potential students are advised to get in touch with the National Bureau for Students with Disabilities, called SKILL (tel. 0800 328 5050); this is open from 1.30 pm to 4.30 pm on weekdays, and its website number is <www.skill.org.uk.>. Help is also available from the British Dyslexia Association; the telephone number of their Helpline is 0118 966 8271 and of their Administration 0118 966 2677. Their website number is <www.bda-dyslexia.org.co>.

---

* Some dyslexic students have objected to being referred to as 'disabled' on the grounds that dyslexia is not a disability. Our advice to them is that they should regard the expression 'Disabled Students' Allowance' as a kind of legal fiction the aim of which is to ensure that they are not deprived of the help to which they are entitled.

Chapter 19
A pianist's story

GILL BACKHOUSE

> Why am I so keen to play music to people? The answer is simple now – and it's not just a case of the musical mind. Everyone needs and wants to communicate with the human beings around him or her. As a dyslexic my words cannot often enough say what I want them to say. Only my music – which I can now see comes from other quarters of the brain – can express the feelings that I cannot put words to.

Thus wrote a professional musician (PM) some months after discovering, when 36 years old, that she was severely dyslexic.

Following a chance conversation about music and dyslexia, she had sought psychological assessment and embarked on a disturbing but ultimately rewarding period of personal discovery. It had not occurred to her before this time that the sight-reading and memory difficulties that she encountered as a pianist were connected to earlier struggles at school. During the following year PM tried to understand her strengths and weaknesses as a musician from a psychological point of view. We had long discussions about her insights as she tried various ways to make the learning of new pieces more efficient and secure. She is keen to share her story, hoping that it will help other musicians encountering similar problems. She prefers to remain anonymous, fearing that in the highly competitive world of professional music the stigma of 'imperfection' might adversely affect her career, or at least annoy her agent!

PM's background is typical of those bright and gifted dyslexics who have shown extraordinary motivation to succeed. Learning to read and write was a struggle, still requiring conscious effort even at the age of 14, although she excelled at maths and drawing. Realizing that she was being 'written off' in terms of O-levels and a professional future, she became determined to prove herself, especially to her academic family. To everyone's amazement she passed O-levels, then A-levels, followed by an engineering degree.

From an early age PM was obsessed by the piano and wearied her family with long, loud sessions at the keyboard. She is quite sure that her musical potential was not evident at this stage. Lessons with her first teacher became an ordeal, as traditional methods of teaching musical notation failed to work. Forty years later she could still recall the frustration of being restricted to plain little pieces, too dull for her musical mind. Lessons were eventually stopped, and for several years PM played as best she could, until another teacher was engaged when she was in her early teens. Young and inexperienced, less sure of 'the right way' to teach, he tried to explain and guide as they went along, letting PM take the lead. This proved a more successful way to teach her, and by the time she was 18 she had passed her Grade VIII.

The extraordinary will-power displayed by this teenager in achieving both educational and musical success in four short years fuelled prodigious efforts on two fronts at once for another three. She gained a performance diploma on the piano in her second year at university and says she will never forget the effort and application required at that time. As a graduate she felt she had finally proved herself, and, inspired by a teacher who described her as a 'late developer', felt free to pursue her most cherished ambition – to become a professional musician.

She studied piano performance for two more years in London with the help of an Arts Council scholarship. She then secured her first full-time appointment as a pianist in an opera company. However, the constant strain of learning new music quickly and playing on demand took its toll. The effort of trying to sort out the score frequently resulted in wooden, faltering, or inaccurate playing, although when she knew the music well her musicality shone through to the delight of the soloists whom she accompanied. She concluded that a career so dependent on sight-reading was not a realistic option and bravely decided to pursue a more solitary path where she could work in her own way and time. It was thus that the concert platform became her goal.

For the next eight years, while supporting herself by teaching, PM studied the solo piano repertoire. Her tutor was a well-known pianist to whom she feels a great debt of gratitude. He seemed to understand the way in which she learned and he adapted his approach to suit her. She was already aware that the way she perceived music was quite different from that of many colleagues. She saw patterns and shapes in music, of which – to her surprise – other musicians seemed largely unaware. Her mentor encouraged her to focus on structure and use the 'architecture' of the music as a starting point. Decoding the score had never become automatic enough to allow her to focus on the music rather than the notes. He therefore encouraged her to study the score of a new piece away from the keyboard as a first step. This intensely intellectual appraisal could take two weeks. The second stage was to work out all the fingering in great detail. He taught her to play with her eyes closed, or with the keyboard screened, and to rely a great deal on motor memory – to trust her fingers and spatial awareness. Under his tutelage, PM gradually built up her reputation as a soloist and has now played for many years at well-known concert halls in the UK and in Europe.

However, the difficulties that she encountered when learning new music persisted, as did lapses of memory. The continual stress, despite all her accomplishments, of striving to develop and maintain her career and reputation was more than evident when we first met. Having recounted her life story, she sighed and said 'Well, it's not much of a success story, is it?' Clearly, low self-esteem had been a terrible consequence of dyslexic problems that had not been recognized or understood. It seemed that neither PM nor her parents had known whether she was bright but wayward, or backward. They had not supported her endeavours or valued her achievements as a musician and this was clearly a painful area for her.

Diagnostic assessment revealed PM to be highly intelligent, with a Full Scale IQ in the 'Superior' range (the top 2% of the general population). She showed outstandingly good non-verbal reasoning but very poor short-term memory. Her literacy skills, by this time, were quite reasonable, although she found reading tiring and made minor spelling mistakes when writing. Testing also uncovered significant phonological difficulties – that is, trouble with processing the sounds of words (but no problems with learning their meaning). This cardinal feature of the most common type of dyslexia had clearly been at the root of PM's literacy difficulties and was evident in her speech too. She stuttered as she searched for the words to express herself, misused words, left sentences unfinished and used gesture a good deal. The *'highly intelligent severely dyslexic'* diagnosis meant a great deal to PM. Yes, she did need to be told she was bright. Learning had been such a struggle for so long that she was sure that hard work, rather than ability, had produced results. As for the dyslexia, it explained her problems with speech and literacy. Now we needed to consider the implications for her as a musician. We found that the book by Sloboda (1985), *The Musical Mind,* gave much food for thought and discussion.

Understanding how a specifically linguistic deficit could have such an impact on initial learning of musical notation seemed straightforward, because words are used to translate the symbols on the page into the many aspects of the music represented by the score – notes, key, harmony, rhythm, tempo, and so on. For example, the link between letter names, mnemonics (FACE and so forth) and music making must be hard for a dyslexic child to perceive. PM was aware of an unfortunate tendency to call notes by the wrong name when teaching, much to the confusion of her students. She immediately resolved to *show* the correct note(s) on the keyboard, rather than tell her pupils what to play! Verbal mediation continues to play a key role in interpretation of a score, although awareness of this increasingly fast and automatic 'double decoding' fades with mastery of sight-reading. PM's ability to decode long and complex scores, even after so many years of toil, was (and is) still not sufficiently fluent to support her level of performance. In short, she cannot sight-read at the rate she can play. She thus finds it unhelpful to refer to the score while rehearsing – 'It is a distraction that gets in the way of the music.'

Her problem with remembering music is to do with accuracy, not with the deeper levels of musical ideas and themes. The music is always 'there' even if the notes are not. The effort she puts into studying the score ensures that this is so. A critical factor that affects her memory is the tuning of the piano. She seems excessively sensitive to pitch and is so upset by slipping tension on the strings that she has her own piano tuned every three weeks. If there is the slightest discrepancy between what she hears and what she expects to hear, her recall seems to be adversely affected. (She is constantly amazed that other pianists seem much less affected by poorly tuned pianos.) Unable to use the score as an aid, she is wholly dependent on her memory of the sound patterns in all their complexity and detail, and she is highly vulnerable to 'interference'. Contemporary models of working memory, which include feedback loops between its subsystems, the stored knowledge base, and the perception and interpretation of incoming signals, seem to support our hypothesis.

PM has many times described her need to prise the music from the page and form her own *template*. She talks in highly graphic terms about having a clear picture of each composition – perceived as a journey through a three-dimensional landscape of structures, milestones, landmarks and colours. She needs to play each piece at speed, hands together, while learning it. In this way she preserves her image of the whole piece from beginning to end. She finds working on right and left hands separately and slowly is fatal – the picture is fragmented and the template disappears. She is clearly a person who needs to work from the 'big picture' (in direct contrast to the way in which most musicians approach the essentially hierarchical organization of a new piece of music – notes to phrases, to phrase groups and finally the composition's musical form). She says that rhythms 'lock into' the spatial form of a piece – only the notes 'slip'. However, 'As long as I know where I am in a piece, I can carry on'.

A neuropsychological approach helped PM to understand her learning style. Given her speech and literacy problems, there is every reason to suppose that PM has a functional deficit in the language area of the left hemisphere of her brain (Shaywitz, 1996). Many gifted dyslexic individuals are thought to be right-hemisphere dominant (West, 1997), having strengths on the side of the brain that perceives form and that codes its sensory input in terms of images rather than words. This 'mute' hemisphere is primarily an organ of visual/spatial processing and pattern recognition and is the locus of much emotional perception and response. Furthermore, neuroscientists have shown that many fundamental musical abilities are processed here (Robertson, 1996; Sloboda, 1985).

Such information elated PM because being 'right-hemisphere dominant' made much sense to her:

> There is no doubt that I've improved my understanding of my personal learning processes considerably. Now I know that I'm aiming to form a right hemisphere image,

it is much easier to bring things together. I have far greater confidence; in fact I am quite excited. In many ways, I'm better, much better than I used to think I was. I've found how my mind works and am able to function on that wavelength.

Several years later, when preparing this chapter, I met PM and we discussed her current views on the main issues facing a pianist who is dyslexic and her own solutions. She feels there are four central issues to be considered: self-awareness, technique, sight-reading, and learning new music.

Self-awareness

To succeed as a performer it is essential to identify and develop one's own individual learning style and strengths as a musician and not worry that others have different talents and ways of learning. To face up to, come to terms with, and overcome weaknesses requires huge reserves of drive and determination – plus the capacity to cope with criticism. This should fuel one's spirit, not damp it down! Good health, adequate rest and relaxation and knowing how to pace oneself are key factors. If real fatigue sets in and too much new music is taken on, one risks sounding ill-prepared, whereas the non-dyslexic soloist might merely lose some sparkle.

Technique

Motor skills and motor memory are vitally important. Perfect control stems from the development of highly refined finger movements, with a small curve in each finger and constant contact with the keyboard. The keys should be *hugged* – 'attacking' or flamboyant styles where fingers or arms are lifted high are ill-advised. Much time must be spent on planning and writing fingering on the score: this links the distances and patterns on the keyboard with PM's own image of the music. The goal must be to move round the keyboard at will *without looking* – to trust the motor skills and memory. Reading the score is arduous but essential when learning a piece or checking for accuracy, so the eyes must stay on the music. Allowing them to shift between score and keyboard leads to hesitant rhythms and is avoided by practising with the lid propped half open. This is a particularly valuable method when learning contrapuntal music where it is essential that each voice is tracked and melodically shaped. For PM, Bach – indeed all Baroque music – remains a high mountain to climb. Once a piece is known and can be played fluently PM finds it helpful to put a mirror on the music desk to 'pin down' her eyes in the same way as her fingers are bound to the keyboard. She then finds she can listen to what she is playing in a more focused way.

Sight-reading

Presumably this is the universal and major problem for dyslexic musicians, but if one aspires to a career in classical music the need to read music accurately is crucial. This is and will always be hard work and necessitates an extremely conscientious approach. Accuracy must be checked over and over again, a hard task for those who process scores slowly. The contrast between this and playing for pleasure, improvizing and extemporizing at the keyboard – as in jazz – is stark. PM says that if she 'let herself go' she would lose ground and never have the discipline to go back to the 'fine art' of classical music, where approximation and guesswork are completely unacceptable.

Learning new music

The strategy PM finds works for her is as follows:

* First, ascertain the deep structure and meaning of the music. Study its form and communicative purpose – is it a dance or march, a song or a lament? Become intensely aware of the harmony, phrasing and shapes in the music by writing them all on the score. Which keys are used and which scales are formed by particular passages? If the bass notes of a section are in a certain scale with an added accidental, write it down. Note whether a passage has slipped up or down a semitone from a certain point. Mark the phrase lengths – these are more important than the notes – and where they are unequal (for example, two of four bars and one of five). Annotating the score in this way is a crucial stage for PM when internalizing the music.
* Work out the fingering for each section on the keyboard in every particular and write it down.
* Play the piece right through, at the correct tempo, to get the feel of it. Then start to rehearse, always playing both hands together, until a very advanced stage in the process. The focus must be on keeping the whole piece in mind from beginning to end.
* When the piece is secure, record it and ask friends to listen. Feedback is important now. Ask if they were entertained or moved and what meaning was conveyed to them.
* The last step is to work on accuracy – to check every single note and rest by playing with the score and using a tape recorder. The music world's preoccupation with accuracy does not suit dyslexic musicians – 'It is our Achilles' heel'.
* The last few weeks before a performance should be used to check and fix the detail and work on communicating what the composer meant. The basic learning must be done well before.

An unexpected outcome of PM's intense reflection on her own learning style has been increased sensitivity to the same factor in her many pupils. Teaching has clearly become a vocation from which she draws both intellectual and emotional rewards. She now sees that each pupil is unique and that 'received opinion' about teaching methods and resources is not always helpful. When first appointed as a piano tutor at a major music college, she was extremely anxious that the authorities would notice her poor sight-reading. However she quickly realized that she had much to offer students. Her spontaneous perception of structure and phrasing in music is a revelation to those long accustomed to focusing on technical mastery – which she scathingly refers to as 'a mere accurate reproduction of the notes on the page'.

All in all PM feels that she has gained considerably from understanding her learning style, her problems with language and literacy, and the impact these may have had on her approach to music. She is comforted by the knowledge that she has many strengths, namely those associated with the right hemisphere of the brain. While heartily wishing that she was not dyslexic at all, PM realizes that in some ways it has conferred unexpected strengths which she now values with some confidence. Forced by her learning difficulty to focus on music at a level *beyond the notes*, she brings an intense musicality to her concert performances, which critics have responded to, praising the 'tonal colours and structural qualities' of her playing. Perhaps her special ability to communicate meaning through music stems in part from being dyslexic. In her own words:

> 'One could find that a handicap could lead to new and eventually more meaningful and transcending levels of performance than before. There is always good reason to look on the bright side of things.'

Chapter 20
A multisensory approach to the teaching of musical notation

Margaret Hubicki

I. Introduction
II. Pitch
III. Time
IV. General observations
V. Coda

I. Introduction

It is widely agreed that in the teaching of literacy skills to dyslexic children and adults a *multisensory* programme is needed – that is, a programme in which learners are encouraged to look carefully at the text, to listen to the words thoughtfully, to touch the teaching materials (plastic letters, etc.), and to pay attention to their mouth movements when they say the words and to their hand movements when they write them.

Many of the same principles apply to the teaching of musical notation – with the additional requirement that the reader needs to co-ordinate eye and hand movements. In this chapter I shall outline some of the techniques for teaching musical notation that I have found useful over the years.

Some years ago these techniques were embodied in a set of materials (or 'kit') to which I gave the name *Colour-Staff*. A revised version of this kit is being planned. In the meantime it seemed to me that it would be helpful if I set out, in the form of a book chapter, the basic teaching principles which underlie *Colour-Staff* and its capacity to highlight, through colour, music's beautiful symmetry of patterning. There is no one way in which to use *Colour-Staff*. My hope, therefore, is that music teachers will be able to adapt its principles in ways that suit the needs of individual pupils. Some teachers may wish to devise their own materials so as to embody the ideas put forward in this chapter. With suitable adaptations *Colour-Staff* can be used with pupils of all ages and at all levels of competence.

A knowledge of musical notation on the part of the teacher will be assumed; the aim of this chapter is to help teachers to 'get across' certain aspects of musical notation.

II. Pitch

a) What is Colour-Staff?

Colour-Staff is both a method and a set of materials. The aim both of the method and of the materials is to help people to read music by linking colour to each black line or white space of the Great Staff's 11 lines and spaces – these encompass the normal range of the human voice. The five highest lines are called the *treble staff* because they represent high, treble sounds; the five lowest lines are called the *bass staff* because they represent low, bass sounds. The line representing middle C floats in between; when used on its own it is shown as a short black leger line.

One of *Colour-Staff's* basic aims is to fix the symbols in the learner's imagination. It provides clean staves which, like the blackboard, can be experimented with, notes being put on and taken off. Another of its aims is to imprint the different clefs on the learner's mind. A further aim is to help the learner to understand the intricacies of notation such as key signatures. It has all sorts of other uses, for instance that of lessening the difficulties for those learners who are baffled – and even alarmed – by the fact that musical notation uses a combination of black notes and white notes on the page. It is therefore a set of materials that can be used flexibly for many different purposes.

b) Colour-Panel

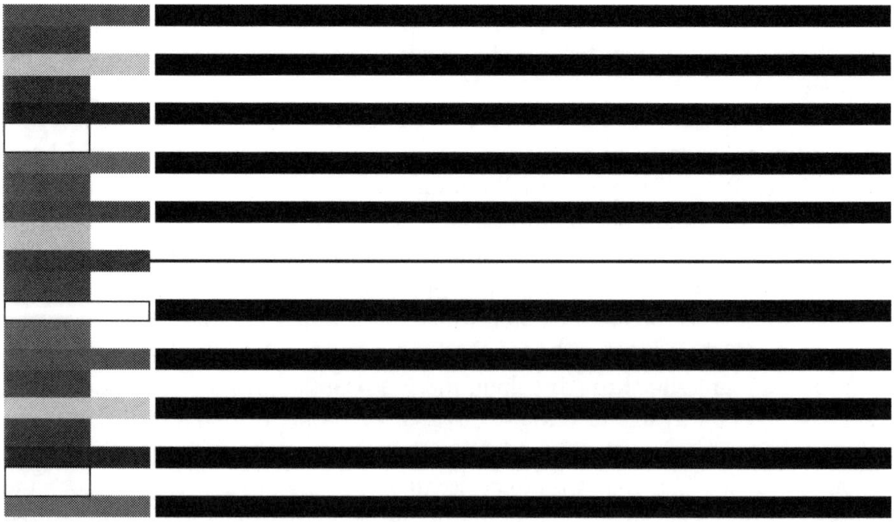

Figure 1. A panel of seven different colours placed on the left side of the Great Staff see Plate 1.

Each colour of this panel represents the name that belongs to each musical sound A,B,C,D,E,F and G. This creates a link which causes the uniform black or white of music's notation to 'come alive' because the learner's eyes are enabled to see

i)   the *place* for each named sound on an instrument
ii) its *position* on the Great Staff. Also, fingers can feel these locations by using *Colour-Staff's* moveable symbols.

It needs to be said straight away that this use of colour does NOT imply any relationship between pitch-sounds and colour – which is a very personal matter. Nor is *Colour-Staff* to be thought of as a 'different form of notation'. *Colour-Staff* is a multisensory 'tool' for helping a learner to focus on, identify, and understand musical details that lie within traditional notation. In some of the illustrations which follow monotone has been used when the original material was in colour. Monotone can be helpful for those who are colour blind. For futher reference to 'Colour blind' see pages 92-93 Figures 7 and 8.

iii) *Colour-order*

Colour-Order	Monotone Order	Sound-Name
Violet	████████	.... F
Blue	████████	.... E
Yellow	░░░░░░░░	.... D
Red	████████	 C
Indigo	████████	.... B
Green	▭▭▭▭▭▭	.... A
Orange	▒▒▒▒▒▒▒	.... G

Figure 2. The order of colours on the panel that represent each sound-name see Plate 1.

Musical notation uses black or white symbols to represent both *pitch-sounds* and *time-lengths* – whether of sounds or of rests (silence in time).

iv) Pitch-Names
The learner needs to know

i)   The *name* of each musical sound – which is one of the first seven letters of the alphabet. See Figure 2.
ii) The *place* on the instrument for each named-sound. See Figure 3.
iii) Its *position* on the Great Staff, line or space, which represents each named sound (see Figure 4). These three basic steps need the learner's own pace for feeling 'at home' with them. Plenty of repetition and revision is valuable at every stage.

For demonstration purposes, *Colour-Staff* uses a *keyboard* instrument (piano, electronic keyboard, harpsichord or organ). The clear pattern of black or white notes that these instruments show provides valuable reference for many aspects of musical theory – helpful for all learners whether or not they play a keyboard instrument. Following the same order of steps *Colour-Staff's* ideas can be adapted for use with other instruments such as guitar and strings (for examples see p. 91).

1 Square pieces

For locating each named sound with its place on the instrument, *Colour-Staff* provides small, square colour-pieces with one of music's seven sound-names A, B, C, D, E, F, or G printed on each different colour. See Figure 3 for applications to keyboard instruments.

i) Sound-name 'A'

Encourage the learner to notice exactly where 'A' lies within each group of the keyboard's *three* black notes. If they are aware of this, the learners' eyes and fingers can always be sure of which note is called 'A'. This pattern of named sound and its position repeats right across the keyboard.

The learner needs to understand that although the keyboard looks and feels flat the named sounds are **higher** in pitch towards the *right* side than those towards the *left* side, which sound **lower** in pitch.

Practice games can be invented. For example

Find 'A' in the *middle* of the keyboard.
Find 'A' on the *right* side.
Find low 'A'.

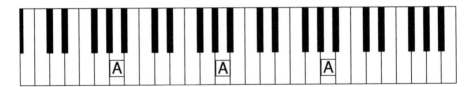

Figure 3. 'A' is printed on each square A-piece. Each 'A' square has been placed upon that white note which belongs to 'A' sound on a keyboard.

ii) Sound-names B C D E F or G

Use *Colour-Staff's* differently coloured and named square-pieces for learning the keyboard place for each of these sound-names. Each one belongs to the next-door note to the right of 'A'. Follow the same learning-steps as used for 'A'.

Continue to encourage the learner to notice where each differently coloured and named square-piece comes in its exact position on the keyboard – relating it to the pattern of two or three black notes, as suggested for 'A'.

While each sound-name and its keyboard position is being learned, endless games should be invented for practice and security. For example:

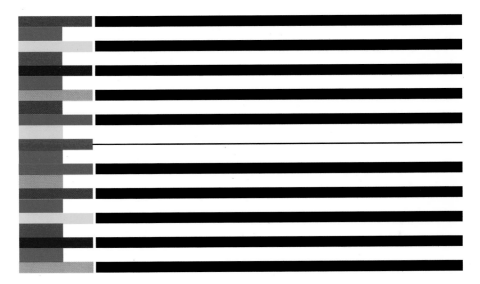

Plate 1. A panel of seven different colours placed on the left side of the Great Staff.

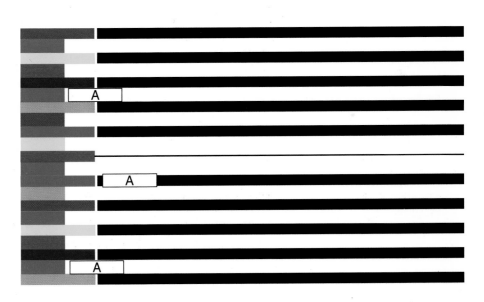

Plate 2. Shows the written place on the Great Staff for 'A' sound-names. By using *Colour-Staff's* rectangles with 'A' printed on each one, the learner will be able to see and, with fingers, feel on the staff that

    1. Sound-name and colour *repeat* at each octave.

    2. Shape (wide space or narrow line) (a) *alternates* at *each* octave and (b) *repeats* again at each *second* octave.

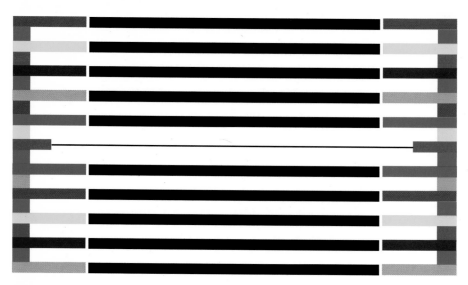

Plate 3. Here the eye can follow, and the finger can feel, the link of colour along the same line or space across from one side of the staff to the other.

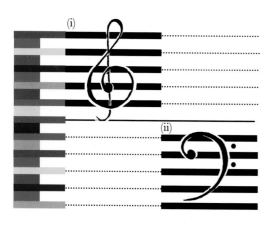

Plate 4. The treble and bass clefs.

Plate 5. Shows the Alto staff (iii) and Tenor staff (iv) placed alongside the Treble staff (i) and Bass staff (ii). These four staves together form the Great Staff.

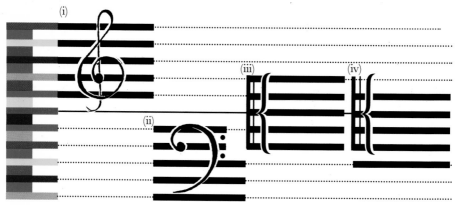
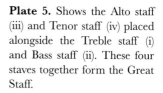

1. Find B on the right of the keyboard
   Find C in the middle of the keyboard
   Find low D
   Find middle A, etc.
2. Is F next to *two* or *three* black notes?
   Does D come in a group of *three* or *two* black notes?
   Where is E? Is it next to *two* or *three* black notes?
   Where is G?, etc.

Constant repetition and revision are vital for learning each name's place.

2 Rectangle pieces

To identify the written place on the Great Staff that represents named sounds, *Colour-Staff* provides coloured rectangle pieces, wide or narrow, for positioning beside the similarly shaped strips of the colour-panel. Printed on each differently coloured rectangle is A, B, C, D, E, F or G. For example, see Figure 4 where the sound-name 'A' is printed.

i) Sound-name 'A'

When trying to read music many people feel confused because the pattern of black

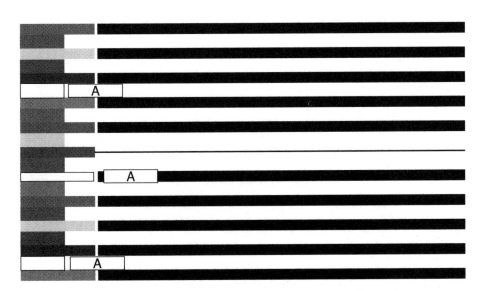

Figure 4. Shows the written place on the Great Staff for 'A' sound-names, see Plate 2. By using *Colour-Staff's* rectangles with 'A' printed on each one, the learner will be able to see and, with fingers, feel on the staff that

1. Sound-name and colour *repeat* at each octave.
2. Shape (wide space or narrow line) (a) *alternates* at *each* octave and (b) *repeats* again at each *second* octave.

or white notes on the keyboard does not relate logically to the black lines or white spaces of the printed staff. Here is the value of *Colour-Staff's* link of colour: it brings out the connection between a) the named-sound on an instrument with its b) written-position on the staff.

It needs to be remembered that on the Great Staff high sounds are written above the middle of the staff – high up – and low sounds are written below the middle of the staff – low down.

Games for practice could include

a) Staff position only
    i) Point to line 'A'.
    ii) Find high space 'A'.
    iii) Is middle 'A' in a space or not?

b) Keyboard location and staff position For example
    i) Point to *middle* 'A' on the keyboard and on the Great Staff
    ii) Show *low* 'A' on the Great Staff and on the keyboard, etc.

ii) From colour into black and white

Point to and name the place on the Great Staff for the rectangle, 'A', as seen in Figure 4 and Plate 2. Example: in the *lower* five lines 'A' comes on the first *space* up and on the fifth *line* up; in the *top* five lines 'A' comes on the second *space* up.

On prepared manuscript paper with a faintly ruled middle-C line, encourage the learner to draw a black oval symbol on each of the same spaces and lines. Write 'A' beside each one (see Figure 5)

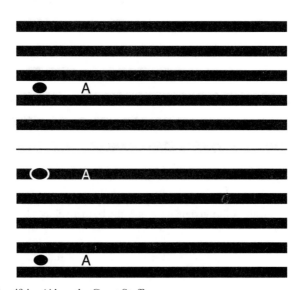

Figure 5. Identifying 'A' on the Great Staff.

By comparing this black symbol picture with the colour diagram (Figure 4) the learner can check for himself if he has drawn black 'A's in the correct places. If not, encourage him to retrace his steps at the beginning of this section and try again. In this way the learner teaches himself to be accurate through his own observation.

iii) Sound-names B, C, D, E, F, or G
To identify the written place for each of these sound-names use each differently coloured and named rectangles. Follow the steps in this section as outlined for sound-name 'A' (p. 89).
    Invent similar practice games

1. Find each sound-name on the keyboard
    Point to it on the Great Staff
2. Combine the sound-name on the keyboard with its
    position on the Great Staff. For example:
        i) Find *middle* 'B' on the keyboard
        Point to it on the Great Staff
        ii) Point to *low* 'B' on the Great Staff
        Find it on the keyboard
        iii) Show *high* 'A' on the keyboard
        Point to it on the Great Staff
        iv) Find *middle* 'C' on the keyboard
        Point to it on the Great Staff

While each sound name's written position is being learned give plenty of repetition and revision as before. Gradually include all the sound-names.
    Make sure that each step is taken at a comfortable pace for the learner – who is then able to pay full attention to all detail.

iv) From colour into black and white
As each different sound-name and its position on the Great staff is learned follow the same steps for translating 'A' (p. 90) into the black or white of printed music – now relating this method to each different sound-name.

1. Suggested uses with different instruments
Colour-Staff's method and materials can be adapted for violin, viola, 'cello, double bass and guitar. Allowing for the different construction between each instrument the steps to be followed are the same as those for a keyboard instrument. Illustrations in this section have not been printed in colour because the choice of the first learning-note to *play* and its written-position on the staff varies for each instrument.

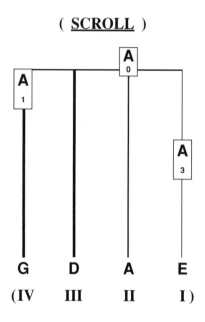

Figure 6. Showing a violin finger board with three small squares placed in first position on the first string E and fourth string G. Each square contains sound-name 'A' with the finger needed to produce it on those two strings. To produce note 'A' on the second string (the A string) an open string has to be played, with no finger needed, as indicated by the symbol 'O'.

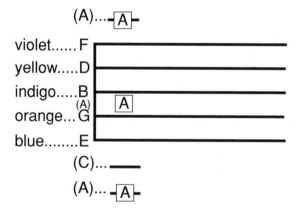

Figure 7. Showing the written position for each 'A' sound-name on the treble staff.

Notice the short black leger lines used for extending the staff to show 'A' above and below it. It will be noticed that each small square on the staff is shown opposite 'A' on the colour-panel (Figure 1 and Plate 1), which represents the written position for each 'A' sound. The print of 'A' causes it to stand out in relief to the other sound-names and their representative colours.

The practice games for keyboard instruments mentioned on pp. 88–91 can be adapted for use with string instruments and guitar.

2. Woodwind and brass instruments

The differences in instrumental construction between woodwind and brass instruments, and the ways to produce a sound, are too varied for illustration here. However, a drawing of the instrumental position for the required sound, its name and fingering could be made in colour, which would link with its written position on the staff. The octave-key arrangement on some instruments might assist the confirmation of patterns – both sound and written. Many recorder players may be familiar with the use of small coloured stickers for placing on the instrument itself as well as on the staff. White ones could be coloured to match *Colour-Staff's* Colour Panel (see Plate 1).

3. Memory aid

If the learner has a problem in remembering that the name of each line or space remains the same straight across the staff, another colour panel can be placed down its *right* side. See Figure 8 and Plate 3.

Figure 8. Here the eye can follow, and the finger can feel, the link of colour along the same line or space across from one side of the staff to the other see Plate 3.

4. Written music

Music is written on five black lines and white spaces selected from the Great Staff.
Each five-line staff has its own particular name relating to its pitch

5. Staff formations

As has been said earlier, high-pitch sounds are written on the top five lines of the
Great Staff, called the *Treble Staff*. Low-pitch sounds are written on the bottom five
lines of the Great Staff, called the *Bass Staff*. (The Alto Staff and Tenor Staff relate
to middle-pitched sounds and will be discussed on p. 95.)

Middle C is seen here as a faint line floating below the treble staff and above
the bass staff. In printed music it appears as a short line called a 'leger' line.

6. Clef

Figure 9 and Plate 4 also shows symbols called 'clefs', which are written at the
beginning of every five-line staff and which name the line on which each one is
placed. To re-check the name belonging to each colour of the panel, see Figure 2.

Encourage the learner to notice very carefully the drawing of these clefs:

i)   *Treble* clef: Inner circle curls around the G line.

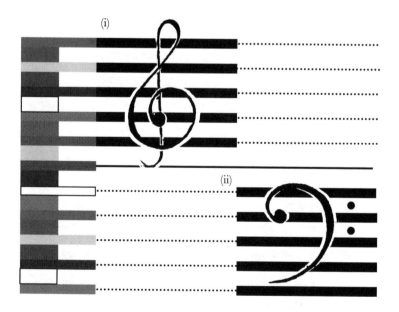

Figure 9. The treble and bass clefs see Plate 4.

ii) *Bass* clef: Dot is placed exactly on the F line – followed by two dots either side of that line.

Both clefs can have two names:

Treble clef or G clef (on orange G line).

: *Bass* clef or F clef (on violet F line).

7. Clef awareness

Encourage the learner to *count up* and, with fingers, feel on which line of each staff a clef has been placed. For example:

is placed on second line up of the *Treble* staff.

: is placed on fourth line up of the *Bass* staff.

8. The Alto and Tenor clefs

Some instrumentalists need to be able to read the Alto clef – particularly viola players – and some need to be able to read the Tenor clef, particularly 'cello, double bass and bassoon players. An advanced violinist who changes to playing the viola may find the principles of *Colour-Staff* useful in making the transition to the Alto clef.

Alto and tenor both use the C-clef symbol placed on the Middle C line, which *always* runs right through the centre of the clef (see Figure 10, (iii) and (iv) and Plate 5.

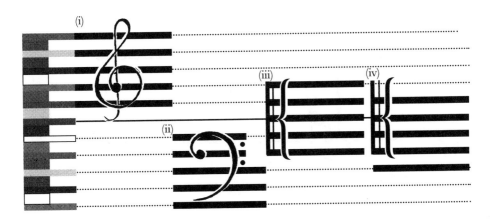

Figure 10. Shows the Alto staff (iii) and Tenor staff (iv) placed alongside the Treble staff (i) and Bass staff (ii). These four staves together form the Great Staff. See Plate 5.

Encourage the learner to count up and, with his or her fingers, feel on which line of each staff a clef has been placed.

- The alto clef is placed on the *middle* line of the *Alto* staff.
- The tenor clef is placed on the *fourth* line of the *Tenor* staff.

9. Colour blindness

For anyone who is colour blind, or who finds music's use of A, B, C, D, E, F and G for naming sounds a real hurdle, it would be possible to think of substitute name symbols for sound-names. For instance seven familiar objects could be grouped in families, as shown in Figure 11 and for this same purpose compare the use of monotone mentioned on page 87.

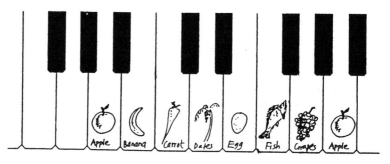

Figure 11. Mnemonics for the names of the keys.

The learner could, of course, choose any objects and draw them as his 'memory aid' – so long as the order chosen is consistent. These symbols could be placed on to the keyboard and drawn on a staff, as in Figure 12.

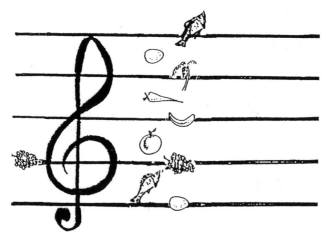

Figure 12. Mnemonics applied to the Treble Staff.

III Time

a) Time symbols

Music uses black and white symbols to represent the different lengths of musical sounds or 'rests' (lengths of silence). Each of them has its own name and meaning. These symbols include:

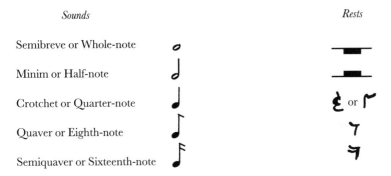

Sounds   *Rests*

Semibreve or Whole-note

Minim or Half-note

Crotchet or Quarter-note

Quaver or Eighth-note

Semiquaver or Sixteenth-note

Figure 13: Names and symbols of notes and rests.

The length of each symbol is reckoned as a fraction of a semibreve, and any learner who has difficulty with mathematics may need special help in understanding this. I have found that coloured counters (or something similar) can be useful for demonstration purposes both for the eye to see and for the fingers to feel – so that students become aware of the different patterns of time.

b) Beat

Each time symbol relates to a regular beat at a given speed. This beat is comparable to the pulse that exists in all of us. People who do not feel a very secure sense of inner beat need special practice in order to develop it. Encourage the learner to listen to the tick of a clock – and then to try to imitate its regular 'tick'.

Say words or names and then clap them, for example:

• a one-clap word could be 'Cat'
• a two-clap name could be 'Mary'
• a three-clap name could be 'Jonathan'
• a four-clap name could be 'Arabella'

Listen to the lengths of other sounds. Imitate them or clap them. Anything that stimulates an awareness of a beat is helpful – walking, marching or dancing, etc. Also encourage the learner to become aware of the 'feel of both eye and finger' following time symbols from left to right across the page (see Figure 14). Fingers should feel each crotchet moving in the direction of the arrow.

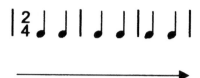

Figure 14. Music 'flows' in the direction of the arrows.

This eye and finger 'awareness' as an important part of learning to read music.

c) Bar lines
Written music groups bars together by using short black lines that are called 'bar lines'. The space between two successive bar lines is called a *bar*.

d) Time signature
The number of beats in a bar, and the length of each, is told by a time signature placed at the beginning of a piece or section of it (see Figure 15).

i)   The top figure tells the number of beats in a bar.
ii) The lower figure tells what kind of note occupies each beat.

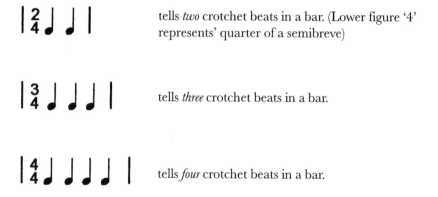

Figure 15. Time signatures.

IV. General Observations

a) Words
It needs to be stressed that words that have more than one meaning or are used for different purposes can cause confusion. For example:
High or *low* can both refer to
(a) Sound pitch and
(b) Position on (i) the Staff or (ii) the Keyboard.

Right or *left* can refer to direction
(a) on the keyboard, or
(b) on written music.

Hand movements can be valuable for showing these different directions. Train the pupil's eyes to follow these movements.

A learner sometimes feels confused when trying to explain what he has not understood or what he means to say – and may need sympathetic help and encouragement towards doing so.

b) Alternative words
When there are alternative words for an item such as

(i) 'Treble' or 'G' clef
(ii) 'Crotchet' or 'Quarter-note'
Use only *one* of each while the item is being learned.

(c) Alternative spelling of words
Leger lines – ledger lines.

d) Colour-Staff Material
Colour-Staff originally consisted of small magnetic moveable pieces for placing on metal staff-boards or keyboards.

The second edition incorporated 'craylux' on cardboard 'Staff-Boards' and 'Dummy Keyboards' on to which small plastic symbols adhere when pressed firmly.

All the ideas mentioned in this chapter could be adapted by using different types of material now on the market. Colour pencils could be used for drawing the diagrams. Alternatively, anyone who likes making things could create small models of different symbols. Small coloured stickers can be helpful for many purposes.

The original material included black and white symbols, numbers both large and small, all of which can be used to form scales, arpeggios, key-signatures, intervals, triads, figured bass, etc.

The small, square colour-pieces are useful for focusing upon both visual and tactile detail. They can be helpful in the early stages of learning:

(a) for building different patterns of colour-order
(b) for placing the first seven notes of the alphabet in different positions:

i) Horizontal
    A B C D E F G

ii) Vertical   G
                                          F
                                          E
                                          D
                                          C
                                          B
                                          A

Encourage the learner to 'feel in the fingers' these two order patterns that the eyes see.

For more advanced work these small colour-pieces can be used to show

a) the *tonic* of a scale;
b) the *root* of a triad, etc.

The coloured rectangles can be used to show leger lines above or below a staff.

V. Coda

Colour has been used in written music for hundreds of years. For example, in *written* music some early manuscripts represent 'C' by a red line, while on the harp the C-string is red and the F-string is black or dark blue.

As regards musical theory, *Colour-Staff's* method and material is flexible and adaptable for individual purposes. It is of use whenever the emphasis is on identifying and relating the beautiful symmetry of patterns that lie within music.

Chapter 21
Gathering the threads

TR MILES AND JOHN WESTCOMBE

Editing this book has been an enriching yet salutary experience. Our colleagues have called attention to a whole range of important issues. In what follows we shall highlight a small number of these.

With regard to Chapter 1, although there is still much that remains to be discovered, it is now clear that dyslexia exists as an identifiable syndrome – that is, as a family or cluster of manifestations that form a coherent pattern. To claim that dyslexia is a syndrome is not to say anything new (compare Critchley, 1970, 1981; Naidoo, 1972). What is new is that recent brain research has put the matter beyond any reasonable doubt (for a review of the evidence see Galaburda, 1999).

Chapter 2 poses many challenges. A central characteristic of musical notation is that it conveys a large amount of information within a small space. It is therefore not surprising that those – especially dyslexics – who for constitutional reasons can process information only slowly should initially find sight-reading difficult. What is striking, as is clear throughout the book, is the wide range of strategies that musical dyslexics use to overcome this problem. We sometimes read in the dyslexia literature that dyslexics *cannot* do this or that, for instance read nonsense words or remembering long strings of digits. This kind of talk seems to us to be defeatist. If a dyslexic musician initially has a particular weakness, the challenge is to find ways of circumventing it. Thereafter, provided the person shows suitable dedication and application, what was initially a weakness can even end up being a strength.

In Chapter 3 Violet Brand pertinently reminds us of the similarities between reading books and reading music. In both cases the central skill required is that of decoding. Both types of skill can be learned, but in the case of the typical dyslexic they do not come easily. This is why there are reports of children who at the age of 6 appear to be – and are – musically gifted but who thereafter run into trouble over musical notation.

In Chapter 4 Annemarie Sand makes a crucial point when she says that 'You really "learn how to learn" only from doing it, not by talking about it.' There are many such situations in life – and not only in those situations relating to music. She also reminds us that, contrary to what might be supposed, singing in a foreign language is possible for dyslexics. What is difficult is having to read the words (of any language) at speed.

Caroline Oldfield calls attention in Chapter 5 to the fact that symbols to which a dyslexic person has been exposed do not necessarily 'register' first time off. She reports that when she has managed to reach the end of a piece – 'an achievement in itself' – and starts to play through it again, 'I'm seeing it as if I'd never played it before . . . Only with constant repetition does something eventually sink in'.

Michael Lea (Chapter 6) concludes by saying, 'My problems had answers.' Not only is this statement a source of encouragement to dyslexics who are struggling; it also calls attention to an important theoretical point, namely that it is very dangerous to make generalizations about *all* dyslexics because one will almost certainly find exceptions. It may indeed be true of *most* dyslexic musicians that they found sight-reading difficult in the early stages. An interesting feature in Michael Lea's story is that he *taught* himself to sight-read because in his job he needed to do so.

Nigel Clarke's chapter (Chapter 7) is addressed to his son, aged 2½. In his account of his early life there is more than a trace of Hans Anderson's *Ugly Duckling*. It will be remembered that this bird, though out of place among the ducks, later turned out to be a swan! In the same way it seems grotesque that Nigel was dismissed from the Royal Marines Band at Deal *on the grounds that he was unmusical.* This was apparently because of his poor sense of rhythm. He adds poignantly, 'I remember that learning to do military drill was hard. If I was not out of step I would be turning in the wrong direction.' An important lesson here is that 'music' is not the name of a single activity or skill; it is rather that being a good musician involves a range of skills, some of which may be easier to acquire than others. This is true, of course, of non-dyslexics as well as of dyslexics: in both cases it is necessary to work at overcoming weaknesses – even though in the case of dyslexics the strengths and weaknesses tend to be somewhat different. There is an interesting parallel here with mathematics. Like music, mathematics is not a single skill; on the contrary it is possible, for example, to be a highly creative mathematician and yet be relatively weak at calculation, or vice versa. Bank clerks who are good at adding up columns of figures and at doing 'sums' are not necessarily creative mathematicians.

By entitling Chapter 8 'Books are my Friends' Janet Coker gives us a particularly important message. In the past, because of insensitive handling on the part of their teachers, many dyslexic children have come to believe that books are their enemies, whereas Janet always thought of books as her friends because, even when she could not read the words, it was still possible for the pictures to stimulate her imagination. The irony, for her, was the realization that within a sheet of music or a musical score there was some glorious music – if only she had had the skills to decode it.

Paula Bishop, too, in Chapter 9, emphasizes the joys that all of us, whether dyslexic or not, can obtain from *words*. There seems to be some kind of contradiction here, because it is accepted wisdom that dyslexic individuals find 'words' difficult. However, the contradiction can be resolved if we draw a distinction between words as tiresome collections of letters that have to be decoded and words that reveal a magical world beyond themselves. William Butler Yeats and Hans Christian Anderson were both dyslexic (West, 1997; Aaron, Phillips and Larsen, 1988), but both had an outstanding ability to use words to good effect in their poetry and storytelling respectively. There is, of course, a similar distinction between the sounds of music and musical notation (compare Hubicki and Miles, 1991). Those who are good at decoding written words, or learning what a particular mark on a musical score means, may not necessarily be talented storytellers, poets, musical performers or musical composers.

Olly Smith (Chapter 10), like Michael Lea (Chapter 6), acquired the ability to sight-read despite earlier difficulties with musical notation. He finds it useful to use his own symbols and pictures to remember articulation, expression and ornamentation. He also reminds music publishers of the value of differentiating different pieces of music by the use of different colours for the covers.

In Chapter 11 Jacob Wiltshire (who was writing at age 11) has provided a vivid and dramatic description of his difficulties. 'A fuse in my mind blows – something there wants to leap out and start playing a Mozart symphony or even 'Frère Jacques' – at least something. But no! Instead I find myself staring into a piece of paper, trying to work out what this means.' The 'blown fuse' image is interesting because it is something that non-dyslexics can empathize with. If one stares at a written word for a long time, or even more if one repeats the same word orally many times over, it is a matter of familiar experience that the word loses its meaning. One may surmise that for dyslexic musicians the same sort of thing happens more frequently: the observer is confronted not with notes that, when decoded, symbolize actions, but with an amorphous blank mass. However Jacob's chapter, like many others in the book, gives grounds for optimism in the long term. The increased understanding of dyslexia makes today's situation very different from that which existed 20 or even 10 years ago.

In Chapter 12, Siw Wood describes how as a result of insensitive handling she was left with an 'outsized inferiority complex'. Her chapter also highlights the difference – not explicitly recognized by her violin teacher – between music and musical notation. It seems from her account that when she played a wrong note the teacher asked her to *name* the note that she ought to have played. 'I made a wild guess – "B". "No, of course it's not, you stupid girl." There ended my violin lessons.' Because a person is weak at learning names of notes, it by no means follows that they are either 'stupid' or unmusical.

Chapter 13, by Helen Poole, is different from the other chapters in the book in that she describes herself as having 'dyscalculia' rather than dyslexia. According to her account she was 'a bright (A/B grade) student at school', with difficulties mainly limited to mathematics. At first glance it may seem uncomfortable to say that a person is dyslexic if they do not have any significant literacy difficulties. However in Helen's case there can be no doubt that her strengths and weaknesses belong in the dyslexia family. From her account it is clear that she had problems of memorization; for instance when she had to repeat back a line of melody she 'ended up forgetting the start of the piece before it was finished'. During conversation she informed one of us (TRM) that it was not until she was 17 that she finally sorted out the difference between 'left' and 'right'. Such problems are all part of the typical 'dyslexic' picture. In addition her love of music and her musical sensitivity all exemplify the 'positive' manifestations of dyslexia. In everything, therefore, except her relative freedom from literacy problems (which in this context is hard to explain, see below) Helen presents as a classic case of dyslexia.

The story of John and his cornet, as told by Sylvia Gilpin in Chapter 14, is one of ups and downs. One hopes, however, that if John can join up with friends who are also keen on music his talents on the cornet will blossom. For many individuals, dyslexics and non-dyslexics alike, making music alongside others, and not just on one's own, greatly enhances its enjoyment.

The piano tuner described by Gill Backhouse in Chapter 15 had transcribed the number 'two hundred and fifty three' as '235' and was 'whacked' for being a 'careless boy'. Many older dyslexics may recall similar episodes, and one necessarily feels some regret that neither their strengths nor their weaknesses were understood. Inevitably one is led to wonder how many talented dyslexics – how many 'mute inglorious Miltons' – have been lost to the world through lack of opportunity. Philip, the piano tuner, had some consolations: he was 'a bloody good piano tuner', but had he lived 50 years later he might have achieved his ambition of becoming a pianist.

The prospects for Deirdre, as described by Diana Ditchfield in Chapter 16, seem good. Even here, however, we all need to remember the extent to which dyslexic children – and dyslexic adults, for that matter – are at risk. It will be remembered that when she took her first examination she stumbled on the stairs on the way to the examination room and, slipping off the piano stool, became so disorientated that she was unable to locate middle C.

James, the chorister described by Sheila Oglethorpe in Chapter 17, paints what must surely be a self-portrait – and a very moving one. Sam, the hero of James's story, was dyslexic. He confused 'b' and 'd' and he liked being by the sea because 'the sea did not critisize' him. Others did so, however, and in a moment of despair he wrote in the sand, 'I hafe the worLB', 'which means "I hate the world".'

Thereafter, however, James was able to give Sheila Oglethorpe a realistic account both of his strengths and of his difficulties.

It is encouraging to learn from Margaret Hubicki in Chapter 18 the extent to which the music colleges have taken steps to meet the needs of their dyslexic students. This should reassure doubters of the advantages of declaring that one is dyslexic instead of keeping it secret.

The account of the professional pianist, PM, as told by Gill Backhouse in Chapter 19, raises a variety of interesting issues. In the first place, the actual recognition that she was dyslexic, with all that it implied, clearly transformed her life. Such transformation is nothing new in itself (for other examples see Miles, 1993: 180–2). In PM's case, however, the new knowledge had a particularly striking effect. She became aware, in the first place, that there was a connection between the learning problems that she had experienced at school and her present relatively weak sight-reading and memorization skills at the piano. Even more crucial for her was the recognition that she had the imbalance of skills widely believed to be characteristic of the dyslexic – weakness at 'left hemisphere' skills such as memorization and sight-reading and strength at 'right hemisphere' skills such as pattern recognition and a sense of the music as a whole. Whatever the truth about hemispheric specialization, there was clearly a benefit to PM in thinking of her skills in this way.

In Chapter 20 Margaret Hubicki describes *Colour-Staff*. As she makes clear, this is a set of materials suitable for musicians of all ages and degrees of proficiency. It can be used for many different purposes, from showing beginners intervals on the staff (thirds, fourths, fifths, and so forth) to helping advanced violinists taking up the viola to learn the alto clef. Its great strength is that it is *multisensory* and was in fact devised in the 1970s before multisensory teaching of literacy skills was at all widely known in Britain.

Some final thoughts

We can but wonder at the fact that some professional musicians went right through their training without being aware that they had problems with reading music. Many and varied are the strategies that they have used, and many of them suspect, as is made clear by Paula Bishop and Michael Lea, that dyslexia in the performing arts is more common than people have supposed.

Experience suggests that dyslexia occurs in all degrees of severity, although in a particular case it is difficult to be sure to what extent a constitutionally caused weakness can be compensated for by a favourable environment. Rather than drawing hard-and-fast boundaries it is perhaps more helpful to describe some individuals not as 'dyslexic' *simpliciter* but as having 'dyslexic tendencies' or as having a larger or smaller number of 'dyslexic traits'. It is possible that some musicians have such traits even though literacy as such was never a major problem for them. It seems that dyslexia can come in all shapes and sizes. This is illustrated in particular by Helen Poole's description of herself in Chapter 13. Her difficulties with calculation and with such things as remembering dates were severe even though reading and spelling as such presented no major problems. (Or was she straightforwardly dyslexic but had learned to compensate for her weakness at reading and spelling at an early age? It is impossible to say.) It seems we have to live with the fact that nature is untidy: when we try to classify she defeats us by producing exceptions!

In view of the successful careers of many dyslexics, we have been sorry to hear that there are still some parents of young people moving in music-oriented last stages of schooling who do not wish it to be known that Will or Kate is dyslexic – wishing no cloud to be on the horizon lest it affect career chances. However, this attitude fails to recognize the constructive approach of many music colleges (compare Chapter 18) whose watchword is 'we can help if you let us know'.

A theme that has recurred throughout the book is, 'What are the relative advantages and disadvantages of being dyslexic?' Chapter 1 mentions the views of West (1997) who has not only emphasized the positive aspects of dyslexia but has suggested that, now that the 'chores' of literacy and numeracy – spelling, punctuation, adding up columns of figures and the like (all things that dyslexics find difficult) – can be taken over by computer, dyslexics are likely to be more in demand than they were in the past. A dyslexic composer, such as Nigel Clarke, is now free to concentrate on the creative aspects of musical composition instead of having to spend time and energy transcribing notes by hand. According to Gill Backhouse (Chapter 19), PM 'heartily wished she was not dyslexic at all' but was still prepared 'to look on the bright side of things'. Perhaps the last word should rest with John Westcombe, who ends Chapter 2 by speaking of 'this problem – or is it a gift?' Perhaps it is both.

Appendix I
Recognizing the dyslexic child – notes for parents and teachers

A word of encouragement

Dyslexia presents difficulties, and the most important thing in the first place is that these difficulties should be recognized. If parents and teachers understand just what sorts of things dyslexic children find hard they can provide invaluable help, not only by showing sympathy and giving encouragement but in particular by arranging for suitable teaching.

Does the cap fit?

A dyslexic child differs from other children of the same age in a number of ways. These differences are not shown by all dyslexic children and they occur in a number of different combinations. The seriousness of the difficulties also varies greatly. Parents and teachers may be helped to recognize whether the difficulties are due to dyslexia by asking themselves the questions that follow.

If the answer to several of the questions is *yes*, it is quite possible that your child is appreciably handicapped by dyslexia; and in that case the *do's* and *don'ts* mentioned below may be of help to you ('several' means perhaps three or four from each section).

So ask yourself

If he* is aged under 8½ years:

1. Is he still having particular difficulty with reading?
2. Is he still having particular difficulty with spelling?
3. Does this surprise you?
4. Do you get the impression that: in matters not connected with reading and spelling he is alert and bright?
5. Does he put figures the wrong way round, for example '15' for '51'?
6. Does he put other things the wrong way around, for example 'b' and 'd'?

---

* For convenience 'he' is used throughout the Appendix in place of the more cumbersome 'he or she'.

7. In calculations, does he need to use bricks or his fingers or marks on paper to help him?
8. Does he have unusual difficulty in remembering arithmetical tables?
9. Was he late in speaking?
10. Is he unusually clumsy?*

(If he is aged 8 to 12.)

11. Does he still make apparently 'careless' mistakes in reading?
12. Does he still make strange spelling mistakes?
13. Does he sometimes leave letters out of a word?
14. Does he sometimes put letters in the wrong order?
15. Is he still sometimes unsure of the difference between left and right?
16. Are there still occasional b/d confusions?
17. Does he still find arithmetical tables difficult?
18. Does he still need to use his fingers, his toes, or special marks on paper as an aid to calculation?
19. Is it difficult for him to remember the months of the year in the correct order?
20. Give him a string of three digits, for example 5-2-7, spoken at half-second intervals and ask him to say them in reverse order. The right answer is 7-2-5; does he ever make a mistake, hesitate or become confused?

(If he is aged 12 or over.)

21. Are there still occasional inaccuracies in reading?
22. Is his spelling still somewhat odd looking?
23. Do instructions, telephone numbers, and so forth, sometimes have to be repeated?
24. Does he get 'tied up' when saying long words? (Try him with *preliminary, philosophical, statistical.*)?
25. Is he sometimes confused over times and dates?
26. Is a lot of checking needed before he can copy things accurately?
27. Does he still have difficulty with the harder arithmetical tables?
28. In reciting arithmetical tables in the traditional way 'one seven is seven, two sevens are fourteen', etc.) does he 'lose his place, 'skip' some of the numbers, or forget what point he has reached?
29. Present him with digits (as in 20 above) but this time give him four digits to say in reverse order, for example 4-9-5-8, If he is asked to say them backwards, does he ever make a mistake?
30. Does he slip back to some of his earlier habits when he is tired?

---

*Some dyslexic children show clumsiness, but by no means all of them.

(At all ages.)

31. Is there anyone else in his family who has had similar difficulties?
32. Do you have the impression that there are anomalies and inconsistencies in his performance, that he is bright in some ways but seems to have a complete or partial 'block' in others of an apparently inexplicable sort?

If, for most of these questions, you feel the answer is 'not particularly' then he is probably not dyslexic. If, however, you feel that some of these descriptions fit him then it is quite likely that he is dyslexic. If he is dyslexic, here are some *dos* and *don't*, which may be of help:

1. *Don't* simply brand him as lazy or careless.
2. *Don't* make invidious comparisons with others in his family or with others in his class at school.
3. *Don't* put pressure on him in such a way that he becomes frightened of failing or of letting you down.
4. *Don't*, without his consent, expect him to read out loud to others.
5. *Don't* expect him to learn the spelling of a word by writing it out a few times in the hope that he will remember it; he almost certainly won't!
6. *Don't* be surprised if he tires easily or becomes discouraged.
7. *Don't* be surprised if his handwriting is untidy and irregular; writing is very hard work for him.
8. *Don't* be surprised if his performance is incongruous; that is, if he manages all right on one occasion and not on another.
9. *Don't* just tell him to 'try harder'.
10. *Do* encourage him in the things that he can do well.
11. *Do* read aloud to him.
12. *Do* express appreciation for effort (for example, commend him for attempting to write a story and, even if he has made many spelling mistakes, remind him that he has spelled plenty of the words correctly).
13. *Do* encourage him to look at words in detail, a few letters at a time.
14. *Do* discuss frankly with him the things that he finds difficult.
15. *Do* help him to recognize that there are plenty of things that he can do well.
16. *Do* encourage him to go slowly and to take his time.
17. (Most important.) *Do* arrange special teaching for him (if possible on a one-to-one basis) by someone who knows about dyslexia.

Appendix II
Checklist of dyslexic symptoms in adults

Read through the list below, Mark a tick for 'yes', a cross for 'no', a '?' for 'sometimes' and 'OK' for 'This is no longer a problem for me.'

1. Do you find it hard to give directions involving 'left' and 'right'?
2. Do you have difficulty in taking messages and in passing them on correctly?
3. Is it hard for you to remember several instructions at once?
4. Do you sometimes get 'tied up' when you say long words?
5. Do you have problems recalling everyday words?
6. Is there a slight delay between *hearing* something and *understanding* it?
7. Do you sometimes mix up dates and times?
8. Do you sometimes fail to remember appointments?
9. Do you ever put numbers in the wrong order, for instance when dialling telephone numbers?
10. Do you find it hard to work out sums in your head?
11. Can you recite the months of the year fluently forwards and backwards?
12. Does your spelling get worse if someone is watching you?
13. Do you still have to think about getting letters the wrong way round, for example b/d?
14. When writing a word do you sometimes jumble the order of the letters?
15. Do you sometimes spell the same word in different ways?
16. When reading, do you lose your place between one line and the next?
17. When you have read a page and turned over to the next page do you sometimes forget what was on the previous page?
18. Do you remember having problems at school with spelling and reading?
19. Did you find it hard to learn your multiplication tables in school?
20. Do you have days when you find it almost impossible to read, spell, and concentrate?

This checklist does not record the talents and skills linked with dyslexia. If you reply 'yes' to more than half of the questions you may be dyslexic. In that case please feel free to get in touch with Adult Dyslexia Organization (ADO), 336 Brixton Road, London SW9 7AA, telephone 0207 737 7646.

Acknowledgements
The original version of Appendix I was prepared for the Dyslexia Institute by professor T.R. Miles with the help of the late Dr A. White Franklin, Mrs S. Naidoo and Mr G.W.S. Gray. Appendix II was adapted for the Adult Dyslexia Organisation by Donald Schloss and Melanie Jameson, whom the editors would like to thank for giving permission to reprint. Some minor modifications of wording have been made in both Appendixes

---

Note: Appendix 1, which is derived from various sources, contains a check-list of possible indicators of dyslexia in children, along with some 'Do's' and 'Dont's' which may be of use to parents and teachers. The original version of this check-list was prepared for the Dyslexia Institute by Professor T.R. Miles, with the help of Dr A. White Franklyn, Mrs S. Naidoo, and Mr G.W.S. Gray. Appendix II is a check-list suitable for dyslexic adults. This was adapted for the Adult Dyslexia Organisation by Donald Schloss and Melanie Jameson, to whom the editors would like to express their gratitude for permission to reprint. Some minor modifications of wording have been included.

Suggestions for further reading

British Dyslexia Association (1996) Music and Dyslexia. Reading: BDA.

Douglas S, Willats G (1994) The relationship between musical ability and literacy skills. Journal of Research in Reading, 17(2): 99–107.

Ganschow L, Lloyd Jones J, Miles TR (1994) Dyslexia and musical notation. Annals of Dyslexia 44: 185–202.

Hubicki, M (1994) Musical problems: reflections and suggestions. In G.Hales (ed.) Dyslexia Matters. London: Whurr Publishers Ltd, pp.184–98.

Jaarsma BS, Ruijssenaars AJJM, Van den Broeck W (1998) Dyslexia and learning musical notation: a pilot study. Annals of Dyslexia 48: 137–54.

Miles TR, Miles E (1999) Dyslexia: A Hundred Years On. 2nd edn. Buckingham: Open University Press, pp. 48–52.

Odam G (1995) Sound and Symbol. London: Stanley Thornes.

Oglethorpe S (1996) Instrumental Music for Dyslexics. London: Whurr Publishers Ltd.

Ott P (1997) How to Detect and Manage Dyslexia. Oxford: Heinemann, pp. 247–75.

Skeath J (1996) Music and Dyslexia. Professional Association of Teachers of Students with Specific Learning Difficulties (PATOSS), Information Sheet no. 2.

Vail PL (1990) Gifts, talents, and the dyslexias: wellsprings, springboards, and finding Foley's rocks. Annals of Dyslexia 40: 3–17.

The BDA booklet, Music and Dyslexia is obtainable from British Dyslexia Association 98 London Road, Reading RG1 5AU.

Annals of Dyslexia is obtainable from the International Dyslexia Association, 8600 LaSalle Road, Chester Building Suite 382, Baltimore MD 21286 2044, USA.

References

Aaron PG, Phillips S, Larsen S (1988) Specific reading difficulty in historically famous persons. Journal of Learning Disabilities 31(9): 521–84.

Bille A (1922) New Method for Double Bass (First Part, Book I, ER 261). Milan: Ricordi.

Critchley M (1970) The Dyslexic Child. London: Heinemann.

Critchley M (1971) Talk on Dyslexia delivered in Sydney, Australia.

Critchley M. (1981) Dyslexia: an overview in G.Th. Pavlidis and T.R.Miles (eds) Dyslexia Research and Its Applications to Education. Chichester: Wiley, pp. 1–11.

Dienes ZP (1960) Building Up Mathematics. London: Hutchinson.

Galaburda AM (1999) Developmental dyslexia: a multilevel syndrome. Dyslexia: An International Journal of Research and Practice 6(4): 183–91.

Galaburda AM, Livingstone MS (1993) Evidence for a magnocellular deficit in developmental dyslexia in P.Tallal (ed) Annals of the New York Academy of Sciences, pp. 70–81.

Gillingham A, Stillman BE (1969) Remedial Training for Children with Specific Disability in Reading, Spelling and Penmanship. Cambridge MA: Educators' Publishing Service.

Gilroy DE (1995) Stress factors in the college student in TR Miles and V P Varma (eds) Dyslexia and Stress. London: Whurr Publishers Ltd, pp. 55–72.

Gilroy DE, Miles TR (1995) Dyslexia at College. London: Routledge.

Hubicki M, Miles TR (1991) Musical notation and multisensory learning. Child Language Teaching and Therapy 7(1): 61–78.

Livingstone MS, Rosen GD, Drislane FW, Galaburda AM (1991) Physiological and anatomical evidence for a magnocellular defect in dyslexia. Proceedings of the National Academy of Sciences, USA 88: 7943–7.

Miles TR (1993) Dyslexia: the Pattern of Difficulties. 2nd edn. London: Whurr Publishers Ltd.

Miles TR (1996) Do dyslexic children have IQs? Dyslexia: An International Journal of Research and Practice, 2(3): 175–8.

Miles TR, Wheeler TJ, Haslum MN (1994) Dyslexia and the middle classes. Links 2, 1(2): 17–19.

Miles TR, Haslum MN, Wheeler TJ (1998) Gender ratio in dyslexia. Annals of Dyslexia 48: 27–55.

Miles TR, Miles E (1999) Dyslexia: A Hundred Years On (2nd edn). Buckingham: Open University press.

Naidoo S (1972) Specific Dyslexia. London: Heinemann.

Nicolson RI, Fawcett AJ, Berry EL, Jenkins IH, Dean P, Brooks DJ (1999) Association of abnormal cerebellar activation with motor learning difficulties in dyslexic adults. Lancet 353: 1662–7.

Overy K (2000) Dyslexia, Temporal Processing and music: The Potential of Music as an Early Learning Aid for Dyslexic Children. Psychology of Music 28(2): 218–29.

Pennington BF (ed.) (1991) Reading Disabilities: Genetic and Neurological Influences. Dordrecht: Kluwer.

Reid Lyon G, Rumsey JM (1996) Neuroimaging: A Window to the Neurological Foundations of Behaviour and Learning in Children. Baltimore MD: Paul H.Brookes.

Riddick B, Sterlung C, Farmer M, Morgan S (1999) Self-esteem and anxiety in the educational histories of adult dyslexic students. Dyslexia: An International Journal of Research and Practice 6(4): 227–48.

Robertson P (1996) Music and the mind. London: Channel 4 Television.

Shaywitz SE (1996) Dyslexia. Scientific American 275(5): 78–84.

Simandl E (1964) New Method for the Double Bass (revised and edited by F Zimmerman). New York: Carl Fischer Inc.

Singleton CH (1998) Dyslexia in Higher Education: Policy, Provision and Practice. The Report of the Working Party on Dyslexia in Higher Education. Hull: University of Hull.

Sloboda JA (1985) The Musical Mind: the Cognitive Psychology of Music. Oxford: Oxford University Press.

West TG (1997) In the mind's eye: visual thinkers, gifted people with learning difficulties, computer images, and the ironies of creativity. New York: Prometheus Books.

Index